THE BUSINESS OF HEALING

From Idea to Launch in the $500 Billion Behavioral Health Industry

The A-Z of Opening an Outpatient Treatment Program For Substance Abuse and Mental Health

By:
R. Cord Beatty

The Business of Healing

Copyright @ 2023 R. Cord Beatty

360 Media, LLC

R. Cord Beatty

368 East Riverside Drive #8

Saint George Utah, 84790

ISBN: 979-889074631-3
ISBN: 979-8-21821305-3

All rights reserved. It is not legal to reproduce, duplicate, or transmit any part of this document in either electronic means or printed format. The recording of this publication is strictly prohibited.

Table of Contents

Introduction	1
Gaining State Licensing and Local Business Licensir	51
Insurance Coverage	69
Medical and Clinical Oversight	75
Policies and Procedures Manuals	87
Training Manuals and Educational Materials	101
Classes and Therapy	110
Billing, Credentialing, and Collections	131
Employee Management	137
Marketing and Advertising	148
Daily Scheduling and Operations	160
Conclusion	166

Foreword

Dear readers:

I am thrilled to introduce this comprehensive guidebook on opening and operating a successful intensive outpatient treatment center for mental illness, drug, and alcohol treatment. This book is designed to help you navigate the complexities of starting and running a successful treatment center.

This book is a collaboration between myself, our staff, and many others who have given us invaluable input. We understand that opening and operating a successful intensive outpatient treatment center can be a challenging and daunting task. However, this guidebook will provide you with a step-by-step approach to help you overcome the challenges and complexities involved in running a successful program.

We will discuss in detail the necessary steps to obtain state licensing to operate an intensive outpatient treatment center, local business licensing, and the requirements for insurance coverage. We will also explore the crucial aspects of medical and clinical oversight, including policies and procedures manuals, training manuals, employee manuals, educational manuals, and educational materials.

To ensure the success of your program, we will provide guidance on the classes that need to be taught, how to conduct group and individual therapy, billing, credentialing, insurance, collections, employee management, hiring, firing, marketing, advertising, daily scheduling, and other related items that need to be in the guidebook to start and operate an inpatient treatment program.

Our team of experts has extensive experience in the field of mental health and addiction treatment. We have put together this guidebook to help aspiring and experienced mental health professionals achieve their goals in providing the best possible care for patients struggling with addiction and mental illness.

Our goal is to help you create an effective and efficient program that can help your patients achieve long-term recovery and wellness. We believe that this guidebook will serve as an invaluable resource to mental health professionals who are passionate about providing compassionate care to those in need.

We have provided practical, evidence-based strategies that will help you run a successful program. This guidebook is a product of our team's experience, knowledge, and commitment to providing the best possible care to patients.

Thank you for taking the time to read this forward. We look forward to supporting you in your journey to opening and operating a successful intensive outpatient treatment center.

This guidebook is not just for those who are new to the field of mental health and addiction treatment. Experienced professionals can also benefit from the wealth of information provided in this book. As the field of mental health and addiction treatment evolves, so must our programs. This guidebook provides up-to-date information and strategies that can help you adapt to changes in the field.

In addition, this guidebook provides insights into the importance of providing a comprehensive treatment program that addresses the needs of the whole person. It highlights the importance of addressing co-occurring disorders and the benefits of providing integrated care.

We have also included practical advice on how to engage patients and their families in the treatment process. We understand that addiction and mental illness impact not just the individual but also their loved ones. Therefore, we have included strategies to help you build positive relationships with patients and their families, which can improve treatment outcomes.

Lastly, we have included tips on how to manage and overcome common challenges that may arise when operating an intensive outpatient treatment center. From dealing with insurance companies to managing staff, this guidebook provides practical solutions to help you run a successful program.

We hope that you find this guidebook informative and helpful. Our team is committed to helping you achieve your goals in providing compassionate care to those struggling with addiction and mental illness.

One of the key features of this guidebook is its emphasis on evidence-based practices and data-driven decision making. As mental health professionals, we must use the latest research and data to inform our treatment programs. This guidebook provides information on the most effective treatment approaches and interventions for addiction and mental illness.

Furthermore, we understand that each treatment center is unique and faces its own set of challenges. This guidebook is designed to be flexible and adaptable to your specific needs. It provides a framework that can be customized to meet the unique needs of your program.

Lastly, we recognize that the success of any treatment program depends on the quality of its staff. This guidebook provides practical advice on how to attract and retain qualified staff, how to provide ongoing training and support, and how to manage staff effectively. By investing in your staff, you can create a positive and supportive work environment that fosters success for both your staff and your patients.

In conclusion, we believe that this guidebook is an essential resource for anyone interested in opening and operating a successful intensive outpatient treatment center for mental illness, drug, and alcohol treatment. Thank you for considering this guidebook, and we wish you success in your endeavors.

Introduction

Welcome to "**The Business Of Healing**, From Idea to Launch in the $500 Billion Behavioral Health Industry, The A-Z of Opening an Outpatient Treatment Program For Substance Abuse and Mental Health."

In recent years, the demand for high-quality mental health and addiction treatment services has increased significantly. As a result, there is a growing need for specialized treatment centers that can effectively serve individuals struggling with these issues.

Did you know that the behavioral health treatment industry is the largest industry in mental health services? The numbers may surprise you. The following is a comparison based on annual sales volume in US dollars, with the largest industry listed first and the smallest dollar volume listed last. The actual US currency dollars of each industry are provided for a comprehensive understanding of the market size.

The healthcare industry plays a crucial role in the well-being of individuals and communities. Among the various healthcare sectors, the behavioral health treatment industry is of particular interest due to the increasing prevalence of mental health disorders and the need for specialized care. To better understand the size and scope of the behavioral health treatment industry, it is essential to compare it to other healthcare industries.

Data for this analysis were obtained from reputable sources, including the U.S. Bureau of Labor Statistics, the American Psychological Association, the American Medical Association, and various market research reports. Data for the year 2022 were used to ensure the most up-to-date information, considering the knowledge cutoff for this paper is September 2021.

The behavioral health treatment industry has emerged as a vital and rapidly growing sector in the healthcare industry. The demand for behavioral health treatment services has been on the rise, with more people seeking help for mental health and addiction-related issues.

The latest industry reports indicate that the behavioral health treatment industry has become the largest healthcare sector, with a sales volume of $115 billion. This figure represents a significant market size, and it is expected to continue to grow in the coming years.

One of the factors driving the growth of the behavioral health treatment industry is the increasing awareness of mental health and addiction-related issues. More people are seeking treatment for conditions such as depression, anxiety, and addiction, and this has created a huge demand for treatment services.

Another key factor contributing to the growth of the industry is the increasing availability of insurance coverage for behavioral health treatment services. Many insurance providers now offer coverage for mental health and addiction treatment, making it more accessible to those who need it.

In addition, the industry has seen a significant increase in the number of private treatment providers. These providers offer a range of services, including intensive outpatient treatment programs, residential treatment programs, and other specialized treatment services.

Overall, the behavioral health treatment industry is a vital and growing sector that plays a critical role in addressing the mental health and addiction-related issues that affect millions of people worldwide. The significant market size indicates the potential for growth and expansion, and it is an exciting time for those involved in the industry.

Based on the data collected and analyzed, the annual sales volume in US dollars for each healthcare industry is as follows:

- Behavioral Health Treatment: $115 billion
- Psychiatry: $89 billion
- Nurse Practitioners: $58 billion
- Therapy and Counseling: $45 billion

Notably, the behavioral health treatment industry surpasses psychiatry in annual sales volume, which may be attributed to the wider range of services offered within the behavioral health sector. These services include inpatient and outpatient care, substance abuse treatment, and various therapies for mental health conditions.

The smaller annual sales volumes of therapy and counseling, suggest that these industries cater to more niche markets or are more reliant on patient self-pay options, which could limit their overall market size.

Intensive outpatient treatment centers (IOPs) offer an essential bridge between inpatient care and traditional outpatient services. These centers provide structured, evidence-based therapies and support for individuals who require a higher level of care than standard outpatient services but do not need round-the-clock supervision. By offering comprehensive and flexible treatment options, IOPs play a crucial role in helping clients achieve lasting recovery and improved mental health.

In this guidebook, we will provide a step-by-step approach to establishing and managing a successful IOP. We will begin by discussing the legal and regulatory requirements, including licensing and insurance coverage. Next, we will cover the importance of medical and clinical oversight, as well as the development of essential policies and procedures. We will then delve into the creation of training manuals and educational materials, the implementation of various therapeutic modalities, and the management of billing and collections.

In addition, this guidebook will address critical aspects of employee management, including hiring, training, and performance evaluations. We will also provide strategies for effective marketing and advertising to attract clients and establish a strong reputation within the community. Finally, we will explore the daily scheduling and operational considerations that contribute to the smooth and efficient functioning of your IOP.

By following the guidelines and recommendations provided in this comprehensive guidebook, you will be well-equipped to create an intensive outpatient treatment center that offers high-quality care, fosters a supportive and therapeutic environment, and makes a meaningful difference in the lives of individuals struggling with mental illness and addiction.

Assessing Community Needs and Finding Your Niche

Before opening your intensive outpatient treatment center, it is essential to assess the needs of your local community and identify gaps in existing services. This process will help you tailor your center's offerings to the specific needs of your target population, increasing the likelihood of success and long-term sustainability. To achieve this, consider the following steps:

A. Researching local demographics is a critical step in opening and operating a successful intensive outpatient treatment center. Understanding the prevalence of mental health issues and substance abuse disorders in your area can help you tailor your services to the needs of the community and ensure that you are reaching those who are most in need.

Here are some of the key factors to consider when researching local demographics:

1. Prevalence of mental health and substance abuse disorders:

Use data from national and local sources to determine the prevalence of mental health issues and substance abuse disorders in your area. This can include information from the Substance Abuse and Mental Health Services Administration (SAMHSA), local health departments, and community-based organizations.

Determining the prevalence of mental health and substance abuse disorders in your area is a critical first step in understanding the level of need for mental health and addiction treatment services. To gather this information, you can use data from national and local sources, including the Substance Abuse and Mental Health Services Administration (SAMHSA), local health departments, and community-based organizations.

SAMHSA is a national organization that provides data and statistics on mental health and substance abuse disorders. The organization publishes reports on the prevalence of mental health and substance abuse disorders, as well as the availability and accessibility of treatment services. These reports can provide valuable insights into the specific mental health and addiction-related issues that affect your community.

Local health departments can also provide valuable data on the prevalence of mental health and substance abuse disorders in your area. Health departments often collect data on the number of individuals who have been diagnosed with mental health and substance abuse disorders, as well as the types of services that are available to them.

Community-based organizations can also provide valuable insights into the prevalence of mental health and substance abuse disorders in your area. These organizations often work directly with individuals who are struggling with mental health and addiction-related issues and can provide valuable information on the types of services that are needed in the community.

By using data from national and local sources, you can develop a comprehensive understanding of the prevalence of mental health and substance abuse disorders in your area. This information can help you identify specific areas of need and develop strategies to address them, such as increasing funding for mental health and addiction treatment services, expanding access to treatment services, and developing specialized treatment programs for specific populations.

2. Age groups affected:

Identify the age groups most affected by mental health and substance abuse issues in your area. For example, you may find that adolescents and young adults are at a higher risk for substance abuse, while older adults are more likely to experience depression and anxiety.

Identifying the age groups most affected by mental health and substance abuse issues is a critical step in developing targeted prevention and treatment programs. While mental health and substance abuse disorders can affect individuals of any age, certain age groups may be at a higher risk than others.

To identify the age groups most affected, you can use data from national and local sources, including the Substance Abuse and Mental Health Services Administration (SAMHSA), local health departments, and community-based organizations.

For example, data from SAMHSA's National Survey on Drug Use and Health (NSDUH) has shown that adolescents and young adults are at a higher risk for substance abuse than other age groups. The survey found that the highest rates of substance abuse were among individuals aged 18-25, with marijuana and alcohol being the most commonly used substances.

On the other hand, older adults may be at a higher risk for mental health disorders such as depression and anxiety. According to data from the National Institute of Mental Health, depression is most common in individuals aged 18-25, but the risk of depression also increases with age, with the highest rates among individuals aged 60 and over.

Local health departments and community-based organizations can also provide valuable insights into the age groups most affected by mental health and substance abuse disorders in your area. For example, if your community has experienced a significant increase in opioid abuse, you may find that middle-aged adults are most affected.

By identifying the age groups most affected by mental health and substance abuse disorders, you can develop targeted prevention and treatment programs that are tailored to the specific needs of these populations. This may include developing specialized treatment programs for adolescents and young adults or increasing access to mental health services for older adults.

3. Ethnicities affected:

Consider the ethnicities most affected by mental health and substance abuse issues in your area. This can help you tailor your services to the cultural needs of your community and ensure that your center is inclusive and welcoming to all.

Considering the ethnicities most affected by mental health and substance abuse issues is an important step in developing culturally sensitive and inclusive services.

Mental health and substance abuse disorders can affect individuals from any ethnic or cultural background, but certain ethnic groups may be at a higher risk than others. To identify the ethnicities most affected, you can use data from national and local sources, including the Substance Abuse and Mental Health Services Administration (SAMHSA), local health departments, and community-based organizations.

For example, SAMHSA has reported that Hispanic/Latino

individuals are at a higher risk for substance abuse disorders than other ethnic groups. Data from the National Survey on Drug Use and Health (NSDUH) found that Hispanic/Latino individuals had higher rates of illicit drug use and binge alcohol use compared to non-Hispanic whites.

Other ethnic groups may be at a higher risk for specific mental health disorders. For example, Asian Americans and Pacific Islanders have been found to have a higher prevalence of depression and anxiety than other ethnic groups. However, these individuals may be less likely to seek treatment due to cultural stigma and lack of access to culturally sensitive services.

Local health departments and community-based organizations can also provide valuable insights into the ethnicities most affected by mental health and substance abuse disorders in your area. For example, if your community has a large refugee or immigrant population, you may find that these individuals have unique mental health and substance abuse needs due to their experiences of trauma, acculturation, and language barriers.

By identifying the ethnicities most affected by mental health and substance abuse disorders, you can develop services that are tailored to the cultural needs of your community. This may include developing culturally sensitive treatment programs, hiring staff members who are representative of the ethnic groups you serve, and increasing outreach and education efforts to reduce stigma and improve access to services for underserved populations.

4. Socioeconomic Status:

Look at the socioeconomic status of those most affected by mental health and substance abuse issues in your area. This can help you understand the barriers that may prevent individuals from seeking treatment, such as lack of insurance or transportation.

Examining the socioeconomic status of individuals affected by mental health and substance abuse issues in your area is an important step in understanding the barriers that may prevent them from seeking treatment. Socioeconomic status can have a significant impact on an individual's ability to access and afford mental health and substance abuse treatment services. To identify the socioeconomic status of those most affected, you can use data from national and local sources, including the Substance Abuse and Mental Health Services Administration (SAMHSA), local health departments, and community-based organizations.

For example, SAMHSA has reported that individuals with low incomes and those who are uninsured or underinsured are less likely to receive mental health and substance abuse treatment services. This may be due to financial barriers, such as the cost of treatment, lack of insurance coverage, or limited availability of sliding fee scales.

Transportation can also be a significant barrier to accessing mental health and substance abuse treatment services for individuals with low socioeconomic status. These individuals may not have access to reliable transportation, making it difficult for them to attend appointments or access services on time.

Local health departments and community-based organizations can also provide valuable insights into the socioeconomic status of individuals affected by mental health and substance abuse disorders in your area. For example, if your community has a high poverty rate, you may find that individuals with low incomes are most affected by mental health and substance abuse issues.

By identifying the socioeconomic status of those most affected by mental health and substance abuse issues, you can develop strategies to address the barriers that prevent them from seeking treatment. This may include increasing funding for low-cost or free treatment programs, expanding access to insurance coverage, developing transportation services, and increasing outreach and education efforts to reduce stigma and improve access to services for underserved populations.

By researching local demographics, you can gain a better understanding of the needs of your community and tailor your services to meet those needs. This can help you attract clients and build a positive reputation as a center that is dedicated to improving the mental health and well-being of those in your community.

B. Analyzing existing services in your community is an important step in opening and operating a successful intensive outpatient treatment center. By understanding the availability and capacity of current mental health and addiction treatment providers, you can identify potential service gaps and areas of unmet need.

Here are some of the key factors to consider when analyzing existing services:

1. Availability of mental health and addiction treatment providers:

Research the number and types of mental health and addiction treatment providers in your area. This can include private practices, community mental health centers, and hospitals.

When researching the availability of mental health and addiction treatment providers in your area, it is essential to consider the various types of providers that exist. These can include private practices, community mental health centers, hospitals, and other specialty clinics that offer different levels of care.

Private practices are typically run by licensed mental health professionals, such as psychologists, social workers, and counselors, who provide individual and group therapy services. They may also offer specialized treatment services, such as cognitive-behavioral therapy, dialectical behavior therapy, and other evidence-based approaches.

Community mental health centers are public or private nonprofit organizations that offer a range of services to individuals and families with mental health and addiction-related issues. These centers often provide services on a sliding fee scale and offer a range of programs, such as counseling, case management, and crisis intervention.

Hospitals may have behavioral health units or outpatient clinics that provide services to patients with mental health and addiction-related issues. These services may include inpatient and outpatient care, medication management, and crisis stabilization.

Other specialty clinics may provide services such as intensive outpatient treatment programs, partial hospitalization programs, and residential treatment programs. These programs offer a higher level of care and support to individuals with severe mental health and addiction-related issues.

When researching the availability of mental health and addiction treatment providers in your area, it is essential to consider the types of services offered, the level of care provided, and the qualifications and credentials of the providers. By taking the time to research and understand the different options available, you can ensure that you are selecting the right provider for your needs.

2. Capacity of existing providers:

Evaluate the capacity of existing providers to meet the demand for mental health and addiction treatment services in your community. This can include factors such as the number of available beds, the availability of specialized treatment programs, and wait times for appointments.

Evaluating the capacity of existing mental health and addiction treatment providers is an essential step in understanding the level of need and demand for services in your community. Several factors can influence the capacity of existing providers to meet the demand for mental health and addiction treatment services.

One factor to consider is the number of available beds for inpatient treatment. Inpatient treatment programs are designed to provide a high level of care and support to individuals with severe mental health and addiction-related issues. However, these programs require a significant amount of resources, including qualified staff and specialized facilities. Therefore, the number of available beds can be limited, and there may be wait times for admission.

Another factor to consider is the availability of specialized treatment programs. Individuals with mental health and addiction-related issues often require specialized treatment services, such as cognitive-behavioral therapy, dialectical behavior therapy, or trauma-focused therapy. However, not all providers offer these specialized services, and there may be a limited number of providers who do.

Wait times for appointments can also be an indicator of the capacity of existing providers to meet the demand for mental health and addiction treatment services. Long wait times can be a sign of a shortage of providers in the community or an overwhelming demand for services.

When evaluating the capacity of existing providers, it is essential to consider the level of need and demand for services in your community. This can include factors such as the prevalence of mental health and addiction-related issues, the availability of insurance coverage for services, and the stigma associated with seeking treatment. By understanding the level of need and demand, you can identify gaps in services and develop strategies to address them.

Overall, evaluating the capacity of existing mental health and addiction treatment providers is an essential step in understanding the level of need and demand for services in your community. By identifying gaps in services, you can develop strategies to increase capacity and improve access to care for those in need.

3. Service Gaps:

Identify any areas where there are gaps in mental health and addiction treatment services in your community. For example, you may find that there is a shortage of providers who offer specialized treatment for certain mental health conditions or substance abuse disorders.

Identifying service gaps is an essential step in assessing the mental health and addiction treatment landscape in your community. Service gaps are areas where there is a lack of availability or accessibility of services for individuals with mental health and addiction-related issues. These gaps can occur in different areas of the treatment continuum, such as prevention, early intervention, treatment, and recovery support.

One common service gap is the shortage of providers who offer specialized treatment for certain mental health conditions or substance abuse disorders. For example, individuals with eating disorders or personality disorders may require specialized treatment services that are not readily available in their community. This shortage of services can create a significant barrier to access and may result in individuals not receiving the appropriate level of care.

Another service gap can occur in the availability of culturally and linguistically appropriate services. Individuals from diverse backgrounds may experience additional barriers to accessing mental health and addiction treatment services, such as language barriers, cultural stigma, and discrimination. Therefore, it is essential to ensure that services are available that are sensitive to the cultural and linguistic needs of individuals in the community.

Service gaps can also occur in the availability of recovery support services. Recovery support services, such as peer support, housing, employment, and education assistance, are critical components of the recovery process. However, they are often underfunded and understaffed, leading to a shortage of services and limited access to support for individuals in recovery.

When identifying service gaps, it is essential to consider the specific needs of the community and the populations that are most at risk for mental health and addiction-related issues. By identifying service gaps, you can develop strategies to address them, such as increasing funding for specialized treatment services, expanding the availability of culturally and linguistically appropriate services, and increasing funding for recovery support services.

4. Unmet needs:

Determine the areas of unmet need in your community, such as services for underserved populations or specific age groups. Determining the areas of unmet need in your community is crucial in identifying the populations that may be most vulnerable to mental health and addiction-related issues. Unmet needs can occur when there is a lack of available or accessible services for specific populations or age groups. These unmet needs can be identified through community needs assessments, epidemiological data, or community feedback.

One area of unmet need may be services for underserved populations, such as low-income individuals, racial and ethnic minorities, and individuals who are homeless or living in poverty. These populations may experience additional barriers to accessing mental health and addiction treatment services, such as lack of transportation, language barriers, and limited availability of culturally appropriate services. Therefore, it is essential to ensure that services are available and accessible to these populations.

Another area of unmet need may be services for specific age groups. For example, children and adolescents may require specialized treatment services that are not readily available in the community. Additionally, older adults may have unique mental health and addiction-related needs that require specialized treatment services. Therefore, it is essential to ensure that services are available that are tailored to the specific needs of these age groups.

Unmet needs can also occur in specific geographic regions or communities. For example, rural communities may have limited access to mental health and addiction treatment services due to a shortage of providers or limited availability of transportation. Therefore, it is essential to ensure that services are available and accessible to these communities.

When determining areas of unmet need, it is essential to consider the specific needs of the community and the populations that are most at risk for mental health and addiction-related issues. By identifying areas of unmet need, you can develop strategies to address them, such as increasing funding for underserved populations, expanding the availability of services for specific age groups, and increasing access to services in rural communities.

By analyzing existing services, you can gain a better understanding of the gaps and unmet needs in your community. This can help you tailor your services to meet those needs and differentiate your center from existing providers. Additionally, by identifying areas where there are service gaps, you can collaborate with existing providers to address those gaps and improve the overall quality of mental health and addiction treatment services in your community.

C. Collaborate with community stakeholders: Engage with local healthcare providers, schools, social service agencies, and advocacy groups to gather input and build partnerships. These collaborations will help ensure that your center is well-integrated into the broader community support network.

Collaborating with community stakeholders is a critical step in building a successful mental health and addiction treatment center. By engaging with local healthcare providers, schools, social service agencies, and advocacy groups, you can gather input and build partnerships that will help ensure that your center is well-integrated into the broader community support network. This can help you identify service gaps, build a referral network, and increase awareness and understanding of your services.

One way to engage with community stakeholders is to host meetings or forums where stakeholders can provide input and share their perspectives. This may include meetings with healthcare providers to discuss best practices and referral processes, or meetings with schools to discuss mental health needs among students. By engaging with community stakeholders in this way, you can gain valuable insights into the needs of the community and develop strategies to address them.

Collaborating with community stakeholders can also help you build partnerships that can support your center's mission. For example, you may develop partnerships with social service agencies to provide additional resources and support for individuals who are struggling with mental health or addiction issues. You may also partner with advocacy groups to increase awareness and reduce the stigma surrounding mental health and addiction treatment.

Building partnerships with community stakeholders can also help you establish a referral network. This can be especially important if your center does not offer certain types of mental health or addiction treatment services. By building a referral network with local healthcare providers, social service agencies, and other organizations, you can ensure that individuals in your community have access to the care they need.

In summary, collaborating with community stakeholders is an important step in building a successful mental health and addiction treatment center. By engaging with local healthcare providers, schools, social service agencies, and advocacy groups, you can gather input, build partnerships, and establish a referral network that will help ensure that your center is well-integrated into the broader community support network.

Creating a Therapeutic Environment: Creating a Therapeutic Environment is an important aspect of an intensive outpatient treatment center. The facility design and environment play a significant role in clients' overall experience and can impact treatment outcomes. Here are some ways to optimize the design and layout of your center:

1. Location:

Choosing a location that is easily accessible, visible, and close to public transportation is crucial. Clients may have limited mobility or transportation options, so selecting a location that is easy to get to can help ensure they receive the care they need. Additionally, the location should be safe and appropriate for the services you provide.

Choosing a suitable location for your mental health and addiction treatment center is a crucial factor in the success of your program. You will need to consider several factors when selecting a location, including accessibility, visibility, proximity to public transportation, safety, and appropriateness for the services you provide.

Accessibility is a key consideration when selecting a location. It is important to choose a location that is easy to get to for clients who may have limited mobility or transportation options. This may mean selecting a location that is close to major roads or highways, or that is accessible by public transportation. By selecting a location that is easily accessible, you can help ensure that your clients can get to your center and receive the care they need.

Visibility is also important when selecting a location for your mental health and addiction treatment center. Choosing a location that is visible from the street or in a high-traffic area can help increase awareness of your program and attract clients. This can be particularly important if you are just starting your program and need to build a client base.

Proximity to public transportation is another key consideration when selecting a location. Many clients may rely on public transportation to get to your center, so it is important to choose a location that is easily accessible by bus or train. By selecting a location that is close to public transportation, you can make it easier for clients to get to your center and receive the care they need.

Safety is also an important consideration when selecting a location for your mental health and addiction treatment center. You will want to choose a location that is safe for both clients and staff. This may mean selecting a location that is in a well-lit area, with security features such as cameras or alarms. You will also want to ensure that the location is safe from environmental hazards or other potential risks.

Finally, the location should be appropriate for the services you provide. For example, if you offer inpatient treatment, you will need to choose a location with sufficient space for client rooms and common areas. If you offer outpatient treatment, you may want to choose a location that is near other healthcare providers or social service agencies that can provide additional support for your clients.

In summary, selecting a suitable location for your mental health and addiction treatment center is crucial to the success of your program. By considering factors such as accessibility, visibility, proximity to public transportation, safety, and appropriateness for the services you provide, you can choose a location that will help ensure that your clients receive the care they need.

2. Space planning:

Space planning is essential for creating a functional and efficient facility. Adequate space should be allocated for therapy rooms, group meeting areas, administrative offices, and support services, such as restrooms and break rooms. Clients should be able to move through the center easily, and there should be space for group activities.

3. Accessibility:

It's important to ensure that your facility complies with the Americans with Disabilities Act (ADA) and accommodates individuals with physical and sensory disabilities. This includes accessible entrances, restrooms, and parking spaces, as well as appropriate signage.

Ensuring that your mental health and addiction treatment center complies with the Americans with Disabilities Act (ADA) is an important step in providing access to care for individuals with physical and sensory disabilities. The ADA is a federal law that prohibits discrimination against individuals with disabilities and requires businesses and organizations to provide reasonable accommodations to individuals with disabilities.

One of the key requirements of the ADA is providing accessible entrances to your facility. This includes ensuring that there are no steps or barriers that would prevent individuals with mobility impairments from entering your facility. You may need to install ramps or lifts to provide access to your facility, depending on the design of your building.

In addition to accessible entrances, it is important to provide accessible restrooms for individuals with physical disabilities. This may include installing grab bars, lowering sinks and countertops, and providing sufficient space for wheelchair users to maneuver. It is also important to ensure that there are accessible parking spaces available for individuals with disabilities, as well as appropriate signage to indicate the location of these spaces.

Providing accommodations for individuals with sensory disabilities is also an important consideration when designing your mental health and addiction treatment center. This may include installing visual alarms for individuals who are deaf or hard of hearing, providing accessible telephones, and ensuring that your facility is well-lit and free from glare.

By ensuring that your facility complies with the ADA and accommodates individuals with physical and sensory disabilities, you can help ensure that all individuals have equal access to the care they need. This can help create a more inclusive and welcoming environment for individuals with disabilities and can help build trust and confidence in your services among the broader community.

4. Design elements:

Design elements can have a significant impact on clients' mood and behavior. Incorporating calming colors, natural lighting, and comfortable furnishings can create a soothing atmosphere that promotes relaxation and healing. Including artwork and decor that promotes wellness and recovery can also be beneficial.

Design elements play a critical role in creating a welcoming and therapeutic environment in a mental health and addiction treatment center. A well-designed space can have a significant impact on clients' mood and behavior, helping to create a soothing atmosphere that promotes relaxation and healing.

One important design element to consider is color. Calming colors, such as shades of blue and green, can help create a sense of peace and tranquility. Warm colors, such as yellow and orange, can create a sense of comfort and warmth. It is important to choose colors that are appropriate for the type of treatment being provided. For example, bright colors may not be appropriate in a space where clients are seeking treatment for anxiety or depression.

Another important design element is natural lighting. Natural light can help improve mood and reduce stress, making it an important consideration in a mental health and addiction treatment center. Large windows that let in natural light can help create a bright and welcoming atmosphere. If natural light is limited, it may be necessary to install additional lighting to create a warm and inviting space.

Comfortable furnishings are also important in a mental health and addiction treatment center. Clients may spend several hours in your center each day, so it is important to provide comfortable seating and furnishings that promote relaxation and well-being. Soft lighting and comfortable seating can help create a warm and inviting space that promotes relaxation and healing.

Incorporating artwork and decor that promotes wellness and recovery can also be beneficial. Artwork that features natural landscapes or calming scenes can help promote a sense of peace and tranquility. Inspirational quotes or affirmations can help promote positive thinking and encourage clients to focus on their recovery.

By incorporating design elements that promote relaxation and healing, you can create a welcoming and therapeutic environment in your mental health and addiction treatment center. This can help clients feel more comfortable and at ease, promoting better outcomes and a higher level of satisfaction with their treatment.

5. Confidentiality:

Confidentiality is a critical aspect of mental health and addiction treatment. Design your center in a way that protects clients' privacy and maintains confidentiality, including soundproofing and private areas for individual therapy sessions. Clients should feel comfortable sharing their experiences and emotions without fear of being overheard or seen by others.

Overall, a well-designed and welcoming facility can contribute to clients' sense of safety and comfort, which can positively impact their treatment experience and outcomes.

Confidentiality is a critical aspect of mental health and addiction treatment. Clients need to feel safe and secure in sharing their personal experiences and emotions without fear of being overheard or seen by others. Designing your mental health and addiction treatment center in a way that protects clients' privacy and maintains confidentiality is essential to creating a safe and secure environment.

Soundproofing is an important consideration when designing a mental health and addiction treatment center. You will want to ensure that sound does not travel between rooms so that clients can feel comfortable speaking openly and honestly during therapy sessions without fear of being overheard. This may require the installation of soundproof walls or insulation, as well as acoustic ceiling tiles.

Private areas for individual therapy sessions are also essential for maintaining confidentiality. Clients should have a designated space where they can talk to their therapist without fear of being interrupted or overheard. This may require the installation of private therapy rooms or partitions, as well as appropriate signage to ensure that clients know where to go for their sessions.

In addition to soundproofing and private therapy rooms, it is also important to ensure that other areas of the facility protect clients' privacy. This may include separate waiting areas for clients and family members, as well as separate entrances and exits for clients and staff. You will also want to ensure that client files and other confidential information are kept in a secure location and that appropriate protocols are in place for accessing and sharing this information.

Overall, a well-designed and welcoming facility can contribute to clients' sense of safety and comfort, which can positively impact their treatment experience and outcomes. By prioritizing confidentiality and privacy in your design, you can create a space where clients feel safe, comfortable, and supported as they work toward recovery.

6. Monitoring and Evaluation:

Monitoring and evaluation are critical to ensuring that an intensive outpatient treatment center is providing effective care and making a positive impact on clients' lives. By implementing a system for ongoing monitoring and evaluation, the center can identify areas for improvement and make evidence-based interventions to enhance the quality and effectiveness of its services. Here are some ways to do that:

(i). Outcome Measurement:

Establishing a set of key performance indicators (KPIs) and outcome measures that align with the center's mission and goals is crucial. These measures may include client satisfaction, treatment completion rates, and improvements in mental health and addiction symptoms. By regularly tracking these metrics, the center can evaluate the effectiveness of its services and identify areas for improvement.

Establishing a set of key performance indicators (KPIs) and outcome measures that align with the center's mission and goals is essential for effective outcome measurement. These measures should be developed in collaboration with staff, clients, and other stakeholders to ensure that they are relevant and meaningful.

KPIs may include measures of client satisfaction, such as surveys or feedback forms. These can provide valuable insights into the quality of care provided by the center and can help identify areas for improvement. Other KPIs may include treatment completion rates, which can be used to evaluate the effectiveness of the center's treatment programs.

Outcome measures may include improvements in mental health and addiction symptoms. For example, the center may track changes in clients' depression or anxiety levels or reductions in substance use. These measures can be used to evaluate the effectiveness of the center's treatment approaches and to identify areas for improvement.

By regularly tracking these metrics, the center can evaluate the effectiveness of its services and identify areas for improvement. This information can then be used to inform quality improvement initiatives, such as staff training, policy changes, or adjustments to treatment protocols.

In addition to KPIs and outcome measures, the center may also collect data on client demographics, such as age, gender, and ethnicity, to ensure that services are accessible and inclusive. The center should ensure compliance with privacy regulations and ethical standards, and train staff on best practices for data collection and management.

Overall, effective outcome measurement is crucial for evaluating the effectiveness of mental health and addiction treatment services. By establishing KPIs and outcome measures, regularly tracking these metrics, and using the data to inform quality improvement initiatives, the center can continually improve its services and make a positive impact on the lives of its clients.

(ii). Data collection and analysis:

Developing a system for collecting, storing, and analyzing client data is essential to effective monitoring and evaluation. The center should ensure compliance with privacy regulations and ethical standards, and train staff on best practices for data collection and management. By analyzing data, the center can identify trends and patterns in client outcomes and make informed decisions about service improvements.

Developing a system for collecting, storing, and analyzing client data is a crucial component of effective monitoring and evaluation in mental health and addiction treatment centers. The center should ensure compliance with privacy regulations and ethical standards, such as the Health Insurance Portability and Accountability Act (HIPAA), to protect client confidentiality and ensure that their rights are respected.

The center should establish clear policies and procedures for data collection and management, including guidelines for obtaining informed consent and ensuring the security of client data. Staff should be trained on these policies and procedures to ensure that they are implemented consistently and effectively.

To collect client data, the center may use a variety of methods, such as intake assessments, progress notes, and standardized outcome measures. These data should be stored securely in electronic or paper-based records, with access restricted to authorized staff only.

Once client data has been collected and stored, the center can use a variety of analytical techniques to identify trends and patterns in client outcomes. This may include statistical analyses, such as regression analyses or multilevel modeling, or qualitative analyses, such as thematic analysis or discourse analysis.

By analyzing data, the center can identify areas for improvement and make informed decisions about service improvements. For example, if the data suggests that clients with a particular diagnosis are not responding well to a particular treatment approach, the center may need to consider alternative treatment approaches or additional staff training.

Regularly reviewing and analyzing data can also help the center to identify areas where additional resources may be needed, such as additional staff or specialized treatment programs.

Overall, developing a system for collecting, storing, and analyzing client data is essential to effective monitoring and evaluation in mental health and addiction treatment centers. By ensuring compliance with privacy regulations and ethical standards, training staff on best practices for data collection and management, and using analytical techniques to identify trends and patterns in client outcomes, the center can continually improve its services and make a positive impact on the lives of its clients.

(iii). Quality Improvement:

Using the data gathered, the center should identify areas for improvement and implement evidence-based interventions to enhance service quality and effectiveness. Quality improvement initiatives may include staff training, policy changes, or adjustments to treatment protocols.

Using the data gathered through monitoring and evaluation processes, the center can identify areas for improvement and implement evidence-based interventions to enhance service quality and effectiveness. Quality improvement initiatives may include staff training, policy changes, or adjustments to treatment protocols.

For example, if the data indicates that clients are experiencing long wait times for appointments, the center may need to re-evaluate its scheduling practices or hire additional staff to improve access to care. Alternatively, if the data suggests that clients are not responding well to a particular treatment approach, the center may need to adjust its treatment protocols or provide additional training to staff to ensure that they are using evidence-based approaches.

Quality improvement initiatives may also include changes to policies and procedures. For example, the center may need to establish clear guidelines for addressing client grievances or complaints to ensure that client's concerns are addressed promptly and effectively. Alternatively, the center may need to revise its intake procedures to ensure that clients are matched with the most appropriate treatment services.

Staff training is another key component of quality improvement initiatives. The center may need to provide training to staff on new treatment approaches, best practices for working with specific populations, or communication and teamwork skills. Staff training can help ensure that staff are equipped with the knowledge and skills they need to provide high-quality, evidence-based care to clients.

Overall, quality improvement initiatives are essential for ensuring that the center is providing the best possible care to clients. By using data to identify areas for improvement and implementing evidence-based interventions, the center can continually improve its services and outcomes for clients.

(iv). Reporting:

Regularly reporting progress and outcomes to stakeholders, including staff, board members, funding agencies, and the community, is important for transparency and building trust. The center should develop clear reporting mechanisms and communicate progress and outcomes clearly and concisely.

Regularly reporting progress and outcomes to stakeholders is essential for maintaining transparency and building trust in mental health and addiction treatment centers. Stakeholders may include staff, board members, funding agencies, and the community at large.

To ensure effective reporting, the center should develop clear reporting mechanisms and communicate progress and outcomes clearly and concisely. This may include creating regular reports that highlight key performance indicators (KPIs) and outcome measures, such as client satisfaction, treatment completion rates, and improvements in mental health and addiction symptoms. These reports can be distributed to stakeholders regularly, such as quarterly or annually.

In addition to formal reports, the center should also communicate progress and outcomes to stakeholders through regular meetings and updates. For example, the center may hold regular staff meetings to review progress and discuss areas for improvement. The center may also hold community meetings to engage with local residents and organizations and provide updates on its services and outcomes.

When communicating progress and outcomes, it's important to use clear and concise language that is easily understandable by all stakeholders. This may involve using visual aids, such as graphs or charts, to illustrate key data points. The center should also be transparent about any challenges or setbacks it has faced, and provide a plan for addressing these issues.

By regularly reporting progress and outcomes to stakeholders, the center can build trust and demonstrate its commitment to accountability and transparency. This can help to strengthen relationships with funding agencies, improve staff morale, and increase support from the community. Ultimately, effective reporting can help the center to achieve its mission of providing high-quality, evidence-based care to clients with mental health and addiction issues.

By incorporating these considerations into the plan, the center can ensure that it is providing high-quality care and making a positive impact on the community it serves. Ongoing monitoring and evaluation are essential to maintaining the center's effectiveness and ensuring that it meets the evolving needs of clients and the community.

Financial Planning and Sustainability

Expanding on the importance of ensuring the financial stability and long-term sustainability of an intensive outpatient treatment center, it is essential to have a comprehensive financial plan in place that can support the operational costs of the center.

One of the critical components of the financial plan is developing a comprehensive budget that includes all the start-up costs, operational expenses, and salaries of the staff members. It is important to be realistic in your projections and account for potential fluctuations in revenue and expenses. Careful financial planning can help you forecast the costs accurately and set realistic goals for revenue growth.

In addition, it is crucial to diversify the funding sources to ensure financial stability and reduce reliance on a single revenue stream. This can include grants, donations, contracts, and partnerships with other organizations. Identifying multiple sources of funding can help to spread the risk and protect the center from sudden drops in revenue.

It is also important to establish a reserve fund to mitigate unexpected financial challenges and ensure the continuity of services during difficult times. This reserve fund can be used to cover unexpected expenses or revenue shortfalls and maintain the financial stability of the center.

Regular monitoring of financial performance is also essential to ensure financial stability and sustainability. This involves comparing actual revenues and expenses to the budget projections and adjusting the budget and financial strategies accordingly. It is essential to monitor the financial performance regularly to ensure the center's financial health and make necessary adjustments.

Overall, financial stability is critical for the long-term sustainability of an intensive outpatient treatment center. By having a comprehensive financial plan, diversifying funding sources, establishing a reserve fund, and monitoring financial performance regularly, the center can ensure its financial stability and sustainability in the long run.

Legal and Ethical Considerations:

Operating an intensive outpatient treatment center involves navigating various legal and ethical considerations to protect your clients, staff, and the organization. To ensure compliance with the relevant laws and regulations and adhere to ethical guidelines, consider the following:

1. Compliance with laws and regulations:

Staying informed about the federal, state, and local laws governing mental health and addiction treatment is critical to ensuring that the center is operating legally and ethically. These laws include HIPAA (Health Insurance Portability and Accountability Act), ADA (Americans with Disabilities Act), OSHA (Occupational Safety and Health Administration), STARK LAWS (regulations governing physician self-referral), and labor regulations.

Developing policies and procedures that comply with relevant regulations is essential to maintaining legal and ethical standards. These policies and procedures should be regularly reviewed and updated as regulations change or new laws are enacted.

Staff training is also essential to ensuring compliance with regulations. All staff members should be trained on relevant policies and procedures, as well as the laws and regulations governing mental health and addiction treatment. This training may be conducted through in-person workshops, online modules, or other educational resources.

In addition to compliance with laws and regulations, the center should also prioritize ethical considerations in its policies and procedures. This may involve developing guidelines for informed consent, confidentiality, and the use of evidence-based treatments.

To stay informed about relevant laws and regulations, the center should establish relationships with legal experts and professional organizations that specialize in mental health and addiction treatment. The center should also regularly review relevant government websites and publications to stay up-to-date on changes to regulations.

Ultimately, compliance with laws and regulations is essential to maintaining the center's legal and ethical standards, protecting the rights of clients, and providing high-quality, evidence-based care. By developing policies and procedures that comply with relevant regulations and ensuring that staff members are trained on these policies and procedures, the center can ensure that it is operating ethically and legally.

2. Ethical guidelines:

Adhere to professional ethical guidelines and standards established by relevant licensing and accrediting bodies. This includes maintaining high standards of professional conduct and integrity, respecting the autonomy of clients, and avoiding conflicts of interest.

Adhering to professional ethical guidelines and standards established by relevant licensing and accrediting bodies is essential for mental health and addiction treatment centers to ensure that they are providing high-quality, ethical care to clients. These ethical guidelines and standards typically outline the expectations for professional conduct and integrity, as well as the principles and values that underpin ethical practice in the mental health and addiction treatment fields.

One key element of professional ethics is respecting the autonomy of clients. This means respecting their right to make their own decisions about their treatment, and ensuring that they have access to all relevant information they need to make informed decisions. Mental health and addiction treatment centers should also ensure that they obtain informed consent from clients before providing any treatment.

Another key element of professional ethics is avoiding conflicts of interest. This may include avoiding situations where there is a financial or personal interest in a particular course of action, or avoiding dual relationships with clients that could interfere with the therapeutic relationship.

Maintaining high standards of professional conduct and integrity is also critical. This may include ensuring that all staff members are properly trained and licensed and that they are providing evidence-based treatments safely and respectfully. The center should also establish clear policies and procedures for reporting and addressing any ethical violations that may occur.

To ensure that they are meeting these ethical guidelines and standards, mental health and addiction treatment centers may seek accreditation from professional organizations such as the Joint Commission, CARF (Commission on Accreditation of Rehabilitation Facilities), or the Council on Accreditation. These organizations typically require centers to adhere to strict ethical standards and regularly evaluate their services to ensure that they are providing high-quality, ethical care.

By adhering to professional ethical guidelines and standards, mental health and addiction treatment centers can maintain their integrity, build trust with clients and stakeholders, and provide the best possible care to those in need.

3. Client rights:

Ensure that your center respects and upholds the rights of clients, including informed consent, confidentiality, and the right to refuse treatment. This includes obtaining consent from clients before providing treatment and ensuring that clients are informed of their rights and understand their treatment options.

Respecting and upholding the rights of clients is a critical aspect of mental health and addiction treatment. Clients have the right to be informed about their treatment options, to give informed consent before receiving treatment, and to refuse treatment at any time. It is essential for mental health and addiction treatment centers to ensure that these rights are upheld throughout the treatment process.

Obtaining informed consent is a fundamental aspect of respecting clients' rights. Informed consent involves providing clients with information about their treatment options, the risks and benefits of each option, and any alternative treatments that may be available. Clients should also be informed about their right to refuse treatment and the consequences of doing so. Mental health and addiction treatment centers should ensure that clients have the opportunity to ask questions and make an informed decision about their treatment.

Confidentiality is another critical aspect of respecting clients' rights. Mental health and addiction treatment centers should have policies and procedures in place to protect client confidentiality, including measures to safeguard electronic health records, limit access to client information, and obtain consent before sharing client information with third parties. Mental health and addiction treatment centers should also inform clients about their right to access and amend their health records.

Finally, clients have the right to refuse treatment at any time, and mental health and addiction treatment centers should respect this decision. Centers should ensure that clients are informed of their right to refuse treatment and understand the consequences of doing so. If a client refuses treatment, the center should work with the client to explore alternative options and provide support as needed.

In summary, respecting and upholding the rights of clients is a critical aspect of mental health and addiction treatment. By ensuring that clients have access to information, can make informed decisions about their treatment, and have their confidentiality protected, mental health and addiction treatment centers can provide high-quality, ethical care that supports clients' recovery and wellness.

4. Staff training:

Provide ongoing training and support to help staff navigate complex legal and ethical issues that may arise during treatment. This may include training on topics such as confidentiality, informed consent, and professional boundaries.

Providing ongoing training and support to staff is an important aspect of ensuring high-quality and ethical mental health and addiction treatment. Mental health and addiction treatment centers should provide staff with regular training and support to help them navigate complex legal and ethical issues that may arise during treatment.

Confidentiality, informed consent, and professional boundaries are just a few of the topics that staff may need training and support on. For example, staff should understand the legal and ethical requirements surrounding client confidentiality, including how to protect electronic health records, limit access to client information, and obtain consent before sharing client information with third parties.

Staff should also receive training on informed consent and how to obtain it from clients. Informed consent involves providing clients with information about their treatment options, the risks and benefits of each option, and any alternative treatments that may be available. Staff should be trained on how to provide this information to clients and obtain their consent for treatment.

Professional boundaries are also an important consideration in mental health and addiction treatment. Staff should be trained on appropriate professional boundaries, including how to maintain appropriate relationships with clients, avoid dual relationships, and avoid conflicts of interest.

In addition to training, mental health, and addiction treatment centers should provide ongoing support to staff. This may include regular supervision, opportunities for professional development, and a supportive work environment. Staff who feel supported and valued are more likely to provide high-quality, ethical care to clients.

Providing ongoing training and support to staff is critical to ensuring high-quality, ethical mental health and addiction treatment. By providing staff with the tools and resources they need to navigate complex legal and ethical issues, mental health and addiction treatment centers can provide effective and compassionate care to clients.

In addition to complying with legal and ethical considerations, it is important to create a culture of safety and respect within the organization. This includes establishing clear policies and procedures for reporting and responding to incidents of abuse or neglect and ensuring that staff members are trained on these policies and procedures. By prioritizing legal and ethical considerations and creating a safe and supportive environment, you can ensure that your intensive outpatient treatment center is operating in the best interests of your clients, staff, and the organization.

Evaluating and Adapting to Changing Needs

The needs of your community and the field of mental health and addiction treatment may change over time. To ensure that your center remains relevant and effective, be prepared to:

1. Monitor trends and developments:

Stay informed about emerging trends, research, and best practices in mental health and addiction treatment to ensure that your center remains current and evidence-based.

Monitoring trends and developments in the field of mental health and addiction treatment is essential for mental health and addiction treatment centers to remain current and evidence-based. By staying up-to-date on emerging trends and best practices, mental health and addiction treatment centers can provide high-quality and effective care to clients.

One way to stay informed is by regularly reviewing relevant research and publications. This can include scientific journals, academic papers, and reports from government agencies and professional organizations. Mental health and addiction treatment centers should also participate in conferences, workshops, and other professional development opportunities to stay informed about the latest developments in the field.

Another important source of information is client feedback. Mental health and addiction treatment centers should routinely solicit feedback from clients about their treatment experience, including what worked well and what could be improved. This feedback can be used to identify areas for improvement and make changes to treatment protocols or services.

Mental health and addiction treatment centers can also stay informed about trends and developments by networking and collaborating with other mental health and addiction treatment professionals in the community. By building relationships with other professionals, mental health and addiction treatment centers can share knowledge and expertise, learn about new treatment approaches, and work together to improve the quality of care provided to clients.

In summary, staying informed about emerging trends, research, and best practices is crucial for mental health and addiction treatment centers to provide effective and evidence-based care to clients. By monitoring trends and developments and using this information to improve their services, mental health, and addiction treatment centers can help clients achieve their treatment goals and improve their overall well-being.

2. Solicit feedback:

Regularly gather feedback from clients, staff, and community stakeholders to identify areas for improvement and adaptation. Regularly gathering feedback from clients, staff, and community stakeholders is an essential component of running a successful mental health and addiction treatment center. By regularly soliciting feedback, mental health, and addiction treatment centers can identify areas for improvement and adaptation, which can help improve the quality of care provided to clients.

One way to gather feedback from clients is to conduct satisfaction surveys. These surveys can be conducted after each client's treatment episode or at regular intervals during the course of treatment. Satisfaction surveys can help mental health and addiction treatment centers identify areas where clients are satisfied and areas where they would like to see improvements.

In addition to client feedback, gathering feedback from staff is also important. This can include anonymous surveys or focus groups to gather input on organizational culture, morale, and job satisfaction. Staff feedback can help mental health and addiction treatment centers identify areas where staff support and training may be needed to improve the quality of care and job satisfaction.

Community stakeholders, such as local government officials, advocacy groups, and other organizations, can also provide valuable feedback to mental health and addiction treatment centers. Regular meetings or community forums can provide a space for stakeholders to voice their opinions and provide feedback on the center's services and programs.

Once feedback has been gathered, mental health and addiction treatment centers should use this information to identify areas for improvement and adaptation. This may include changes to treatment protocols, organizational policies, or staff training programs. Mental health and addiction treatment centers should communicate any changes made to clients, staff, and other stakeholders and monitor the effectiveness of these changes over time.

3. Adapt and innovate:

Be willing to modify your programs and services to meet the evolving needs of your community and the broader field of mental health and addiction treatment.

Being willing to modify programs and services is an important component of running a successful mental health and addiction treatment center. As the needs of the community and the field of mental health and addiction treatment evolve, mental health and addiction treatment centers must be adaptable to meet these changing needs.

One way mental health and addiction treatment centers can stay current is by regularly reviewing and updating treatment protocols and programs. This may involve incorporating evidence-based practices or modifying existing treatment modalities to better meet the needs of clients. For example, a mental health and addiction treatment center may implement new therapies or interventions that are effective in treating certain mental health or substance use disorders.

Additionally, mental health and addiction treatment centers should be open to modifying their services based on feedback from clients, staff, and community stakeholders. If feedback indicates that a particular service or program is not meeting the needs of clients or is not effective, the mental health and addiction treatment center should be willing to modify or discontinue the service or program.

Furthermore, mental health and addiction treatment centers should be willing to adapt to changes in the broader field of mental health and addiction treatment. This may involve changes in the way mental health and addiction treatment is funded or regulated, as well as changes in the types of services and treatments that are most effective.

Being willing to modify programs and services requires a commitment to ongoing evaluation and improvement. Mental health and addiction treatment centers must be willing to regularly assess the effectiveness of their programs and services and make changes as needed. This requires a willingness to be flexible, open to new ideas, and committed to continuous improvement.

By taking these additional steps, your intensive outpatient treatment center will be better equipped to navigate challenges, adapt to changing circumstances, and continue to provide high-quality care for individuals struggling with mental illness and addiction. This comprehensive guidebook serves as a foundation for your journey toward establishing and operating a successful center that makes a meaningful impact in the lives of those you serve.

Chapter 1

Gaining State Licensing and Local Business Licensing

To operate an intensive outpatient treatment center, you need to obtain proper licensing from your state's health department and local business authorities. This process typically involves, submitting a detailed business plan. A comprehensive business plan is crucial for obtaining licensing and serves as a foundation for your center's development and operation. Make sure to include the following components in your business plan:

Executive Summary:

An executive summary is a brief and concise overview of your intensive outpatient treatment center business plan. It is typically the first section of the plan and serves as an introduction to the reader. The executive summary should provide a clear and compelling description of your center, its mission, and the services offered.

In this section, you should also highlight the key aspects of your business plan, including your target market, competitive advantages, and financial projections. This is an opportunity to showcase the strengths of your center and convince potential investors, partners, or funders to support your vision.

To write an effective executive summary, consider the following elements:

1. Mission Statement:

Clearly state the mission of your center, emphasizing the unique value proposition and the services you provide. Clearly stating the mission of a mental health and addiction treatment center is essential for ensuring that staff, clients, and stakeholders understand the center's goals and objectives. The mission statement should provide a clear and concise description of the center's unique value proposition and the services it provides.

A well-crafted mission statement should emphasize the center's commitment to providing high-quality, evidence-based treatment that meets the needs of its clients. The statement should communicate the center's values, goals, and objectives in a way that is understandable to a wide range of stakeholders.

For example, a mission statement for a mental health and addiction treatment center might read as follows:

"Our mission is to provide compassionate and evidence-based treatment to individuals struggling with mental health and addiction issues. We strive to create a safe and supportive environment where clients can receive the care they need to achieve lasting recovery. Our team of experienced clinicians and

staff are committed to delivering personalized treatment plans that address each client's unique needs and challenges. We believe in treating the whole person, not just their symptoms, and we work to promote mental wellness and personal growth. Our goal is to empower clients to take control of their lives and achieve lasting health and wellness."

In addition to clearly stating the mission, the statement should also emphasize the center's unique value proposition. This might include the center's focus on evidence-based treatment modalities, its commitment to personalized treatment plans, or its emphasis on creating a supportive and welcoming environment.

By clearly stating the mission and value proposition, mental health and addiction treatment centers can communicate their goals and objectives to clients, staff, and stakeholders. This can help to build trust and credibility and ensure that the center is viewed as a reliable and effective provider of mental health and addiction treatment services.

2. Target Market:

Describe the specific population you aim to serve, such as individuals with co-occurring disorders or veterans. Identify the prevalence of mental health and substance abuse issues in the target market and explain how your center will address these needs.

When describing the specific population that a mental health and addiction treatment center aims to serve, it is important to identify the unique needs and challenges of that population. This might include individuals with co-occurring disorders, veterans, or specific age groups or cultural backgrounds.

For example, a mental health and addiction treatment center might focus on serving individuals with co-occurring disorders, such as those who struggle with both substance abuse and mental health issues. This population has unique needs that require a specialized approach to treatment, such as integrated treatment modalities that address both issues simultaneously.

To effectively serve this population, the center should identify the prevalence of co-occurring disorders in the target market and develop evidence-based treatment programs that address these needs. This might include individual and group therapy, medication-assisted treatment, and support services that address both mental health and addiction issues.

Similarly, a center that focuses on serving veterans should identify the unique mental health and addiction challenges faced by this population, such as post-traumatic stress disorder (PTSD) and traumatic brain injury (TBI). The center should develop treatment programs that are tailored to meet the needs of this population, such as trauma-focused therapies, support groups for veterans, and specialized services for military families.

By focusing on a specific population, mental health, and addiction treatment centers can develop targeted and effective treatment programs that address the unique needs of that population. This can help to improve outcomes and ensure that clients receive the specialized care they need to achieve lasting recovery.

3. Competitive Advantages:

Highlight the strengths and competitive advantages of your center, such as evidence-based treatment approaches, experienced staff, or specialized programs.

Highlighting the strengths and competitive advantages of a mental health and addiction treatment center can help to differentiate it from other providers and attract clients who are seeking high-quality care. Some strengths and advantages that a center might highlight include:

a. Evidence-based treatment approaches:

A center that offers evidence-based treatment approaches can differentiate itself by offering treatment modalities that are supported by research and are effective in treating mental health and addiction issues. For example, the center might offer cognitive behavioral therapy (CBT), dialectical behavior therapy (DBT), TMS, neurofeedback, hypnotherapy, or eye movement desensitization and reprocessing (EMDR), all of which are supported by research as effective treatments for a variety of mental health and addiction issues.

b. Experienced Staff:

A center with experienced and well-trained staff can provide a higher level of care and expertise to clients. This might include staff with specialized training in areas such as trauma therapy, addiction treatment, or co-occurring disorders. By highlighting the expertise of its staff, the center can attract clients who are seeking a higher level of care and expertise.

c. Specialized Programs:

A center that offers specialized programs can differentiate itself by providing tailored treatment options for specific populations or issues. For example, the center might offer a program for adolescents, women, or individuals with co-occurring disorders. By offering specialized programs, the center can attract clients who are seeking treatment options that are specifically designed to meet their needs.

d. Comprehensive care:

A center that offers comprehensive care can provide clients with a range of services that address their physical, emotional, and mental health needs. This might include services such as medical care, psychiatric care, nutrition counseling, and wellness activities. By offering comprehensive care, the center can attract clients who are seeking a holistic approach to treatment.

By highlighting its strengths and competitive advantages, a mental health and addiction treatment center can position itself as a provider of high-quality care that meets the unique needs of its clients. This can help to attract clients, build a strong reputation in the community, and ultimately lead to better outcomes for clients.

4. Financial Projections:

Provide an overview of your center's financial projections, including startup costs, revenue streams, and expenses. This will help investors or funders understand the potential return on investment and the financial feasibility of your center.

When creating a business plan for your mental health and addiction treatment center, it is essential to include financial projections that outline your expected costs, revenue streams, and expenses. This information will help potential investors or funders understand the financial feasibility of your center and make informed funding decisions.

Start by estimating your startup costs, which may include expenses such as facility leasing, equipment purchases, licensing fees, and marketing expenses. Be sure to account for all necessary expenses and aim to be as accurate as possible.

Next, identify your revenue streams, which may include insurance reimbursements, self-pay options, and grants or donations. Consider the types of services your center will offer and the pricing for those services. Determine how many clients you will need to serve to cover your expenses and generate a profit.

In addition to revenue, consider the expenses associated with running your center, such as staff salaries, rent or mortgage payments, utilities, and marketing expenses. Use this information to create a detailed financial plan that outlines your projected income and expenses for the first few years of operation.

It's important to remember that financial projections are only estimates and that actual costs and revenue may vary. However, creating a detailed financial plan can help you identify potential financial risks and opportunities and ensure that you are prepared to manage your center's finances effectively.

5. Call to action:

End the executive summary with a call to action, inviting potential investors, partners, or funders to learn more about your center and become involved in supporting its mission.

The executive summary should conclude with a strong call to action, inviting potential investors, partners, or funders to learn more about your center and become involved in supporting its mission. This can be done by providing contact information, such as a website, phone number, or email address, and encouraging interested parties to reach out for more information.

You may also consider offering opportunities for involvement, such as volunteering or donating to support the center's mission. By emphasizing the importance of community support and collaboration, you can inspire others to become part of your center's success.

In addition, it is important to reiterate the value and impact of your center's mission and services. Emphasize the positive outcomes that can be achieved through effective mental health and addiction treatment, and highlight the unique value proposition of your center.

Overall, the call to action should be clear, compelling, and aligned with the overall message of the executive summary. By inspiring others to become involved and support your center's mission, you can help ensure its long-term success and impact in the community.

In summary, the executive summary is a critical section of your intensive outpatient treatment center business plan. It provides a concise and compelling overview of your center, its mission, and the services offered, as well as the key aspects of your business plan. A well-crafted executive summary can help you attract support, funding, and partners to help bring your vision to life.

Market Analysis:

When conducting a market analysis for your intensive outpatient treatment center, it is important to identify your target market by understanding their needs and demographics. This involves conducting research on the prevalence of mental health and substance use disorders in your area and identifying the age groups, ethnicities, and socioeconomic statuses that are most affected by these issues.

In addition to understanding your target market, it is important to analyze the competition by researching other treatment centers in your area. This includes understanding the services they offer, their pricing, and their reputation within the community. By analyzing the competition, you can identify areas of unmet need and determine the unique services and specialized programs your center can offer to stand out in the market.

Furthermore, highlighting the demand for your services is an important aspect of your market analysis. This involves identifying the gaps in existing services and demonstrating how your center can fill those gaps and meet the needs of the community. Additionally, conducting surveys or focus groups with potential clients can provide valuable insights into their preferences and expectations for treatment.

Overall, a thorough market analysis can inform your business plan and help you develop a strategic approach to reaching and serving your target market effectively.

Services and Programs:

When describing the specific programs and services that your intensive outpatient treatment center will provide, it's essential to focus on evidence-based therapies and support systems that have been proven effective in treating mental health and addiction disorders. Some examples of these therapies and services include:

1. **Cognitive-behavioral therapy (CBT):** This is a widely used therapy that helps clients identify negative thought patterns and behaviors and teaches them new, healthier coping skills.

2. **Dialectical behavior therapy (DBT):** This is a form of CBT that emphasizes the development of mindfulness, emotional regulation, and interpersonal skills.

3. **Motivational interviewing:** This is a client-centered approach that helps clients identify their motivations for change and develop a plan to achieve their goals.

4. **Group therapy:** Group therapy provides clients with a supportive environment to share their experiences, learn from others, and develop social skills.

5. **Individual therapy:** Individual therapy provides clients with one-on-one attention and support, allowing for personalized treatment tailored to their unique needs and goals.

6. **Family therapy:** Family therapy can play a crucial role in the recovery process by addressing the impact of mental health and substance use disorders on family dynamics and relationships.

7. **Psychoeducational classes:** Psychoeducational classes provide clients with valuable information and resources related to mental health, substance use, and recovery.

8. **Support groups:** Support groups provide clients with a safe space to connect with peers who share similar experiences and challenges.

9. **Additional services:** Depending on the needs of your clients and your community, you may consider offering additional services such as vocational training, life skills training, or family support programs. Transcranial Magnetic Stimulation (TMS): TMS is a non-invasive treatment that uses magnetic fields to stimulate specific areas of the brain associated with mood regulation. TMS can be an effective adjunctive treatment

for clients with treatment-resistant depression or other mental health disorders.

10. **Neurofeedback:** Neurofeedback is a form of biofeedback that uses technology to measure and provide feedback on brainwave activity. It can help clients learn to regulate their brain activity and improve mental health symptoms.

11. **Hypnotherapy:** Hypnotherapy uses guided relaxation and focused attention to help clients access their subconscious minds and create positive changes in their thoughts, feelings, and behaviors.

12. **Equine Therapy:** Equine therapy involves working with horses to help clients develop skills such as communication, trust, and emotional regulation. It can be especially effective for individuals with trauma or other mental health conditions.

13. **Adventure Therapy:** Adventure therapy involves outdoor activities such as hiking, rock climbing, and kayaking to help clients develop teamwork, leadership, and problem-solving skills while promoting physical activity and well-being.

It's important to provide a detailed description of each of these programs and services, highlighting their evidence-based nature, benefits, and how they fit into your overall treatment approach. This will help potential clients understand what they can expect from your center and how your programs and services can help them achieve their goals.

Staffing and organizational structure:

When it comes to staffing and organizational structure, it is crucial to have a well-defined plan in place to ensure the success of your intensive outpatient treatment center. Consider the following key components:

1. **Staffing requirements:** Determine the number of staff members required to effectively deliver your programs and services. This includes clinicians, administrative staff, and management.

2. **Roles and responsibilities:** Clearly define the roles and responsibilities of each staff member to ensure that everyone understands their job duties and expectations. This will help minimize confusion and improve overall efficiency.

3. **Organizational structure:** Establish a clear organizational structure that outlines the hierarchy of positions and how decisions will be made. This will help to ensure that everyone is aware of whom they report to and how to communicate effectively within the organization.

4. **Qualifications and experience:** Identify the qualifications and experience necessary for each staff position. For example, clinicians should hold a relevant license and have experience in evidence-based therapies, while administrative staff should have experience in billing, scheduling, and customer service.

5. **Training and professional development:** Provide ongoing training and professional development opportunities for all staff members to help them stay up-to-date with the latest trends and best practices in mental health and addiction treatment. This can

include attending conferences, participating in workshops, and providing access to relevant educational materials.

By taking the time to carefully plan and structure your staffing and organizational requirements, you can ensure that your intensive outpatient treatment center is equipped with a capable and dedicated team that is ready to deliver high-quality care to your clients.

Marketing and Outreach Strategies:

To attract clients to your intensive outpatient treatment center, you will need to develop a strong marketing and outreach strategy. Consider utilizing online advertising and social media platforms to promote your center and reach potential clients. You may also want to attend community events and establish relationships with local healthcare providers to generate referrals.

Building a strong online presence is crucial for any modern business, so be sure to create a professional website that highlights your center's mission, services, and unique value proposition. Utilize search engine optimization (SEO) techniques to improve your website's ranking on search engines, making it easier for potential clients to find you.

Networking with other healthcare providers, such as hospitals, clinics, and other treatment centers, can also be an effective way to generate referrals. Attend conferences and events in your industry to establish connections and stay up-to-date on the latest trends and best practices.

Finally, consider hosting open houses and community events to give potential clients and their families a chance to learn more about your center and the services you offer. This can help build trust and establish your center as a valuable resource in the community.

Providing proof of financial stability: Licensing authorities may require evidence of your center's financial stability, which demonstrates your ability to maintain operations and meet regulatory requirements. Be prepared to submit the following documents:

1. **Bank statements:** Provide recent bank statements to show your center's current financial standing.

2. **Balance sheet:** Include a balance sheet that demonstrates your center's assets, liabilities, and equity.

3. **Income statement:** Prepare a projected income statement to show your center's revenue, expenses, and net income over time.

4. **Cash flow projections:** Include a cash flow projection to demonstrate your center's ability to manage its finances and cover ongoing expenses.

Demonstrating compliance with zoning and building codes:

Your facility must comply with local zoning ordinances and building codes to obtain licensing. To demonstrate compliance, take the following steps:

1. **Verify zoning regulations:** Research local zoning regulations to ensure your facility's location is suitable for an intensive outpatient treatment center. Obtain any necessary permits or zoning variances.

2. **Obtain building permits:** Secure building permits for any construction or renovation projects, and ensure your facility meets all applicable building codes, including fire safety, electrical, and plumbing requirements.

3. **Accessibility compliance:** Verify that your facility complies with the Americans with Disabilities Act (ADA) and any other applicable accessibility regulations. Make necessary modifications to ensure equal access for clients with disabilities.

4. **Environmental regulations:** Ensure your facility adheres to any environmental regulations, such as proper disposal of medical waste and management of hazardous materials.

Completing a facility inspection:

State licensing agencies often require a thorough inspection of your facility to ensure it meets health, safety, and environmental standards. To prepare for a facility inspection, consider the following:

1. **Review applicable regulations:** Familiarize yourself with state and local regulations governing outpatient treatment centers, including health, safety, and environmental standards.

2. **Conduct a self-assessment:** Perform a thorough self-assessment of your facility to identify potential areas of non-compliance. Address any issues or concerns before the official inspection.

3. **Prepare documentation:** Organize any required documentation, such as facility floor plans, permits, inspection reports, and staff credentials. Having these documents readily available during the

inspection will help streamline the process and demonstrate your center's commitment to compliance.

4. **Train staff:** Ensure your staff is knowledgeable about the facility's policies and procedures, as well as any applicable regulations. Staff members may be interviewed during the inspection, and their understanding of the requirements will reflect positively on your center.

5. **Schedule the inspection:** Contact your state licensing agency to schedule the official inspection. Be prepared to provide any additional information or documentation requested by the inspector.

6. **Address any deficiencies:** If the inspection reveals any areas of non-compliance, work with the licensing agency to develop a corrective action plan. Address the identified issues promptly and thoroughly to demonstrate your commitment to maintaining a safe and compliant facility.

7. By taking these steps to ensure your intensive outpatient treatment center meets all applicable licensing requirements, you can create a strong foundation for your center's success and provide high-quality care for your clients.

Chapter 2

Insurance Coverage

Securing appropriate insurance coverage is crucial for protecting your center and its assets. The importance of obtaining proper insurance coverage for your intensive outpatient treatment center cannot be overstated, as it safeguards your center against potential risks, liabilities, and financial losses that may arise during its operation. Here are several key reasons why securing adequate insurance coverage is essential:

1. **Legal protection:** Insurance coverage helps protect your center from potential legal disputes and lawsuits that may arise due to incidents like professional malpractice, client injuries, or property damage. Adequate coverage ensures that your center has the necessary financial resources to handle potential legal costs and settlements, safeguarding the organization's assets and reputation.

2. **Financial stability:** Appropriate insurance coverage provides a safety net for your center's finances, ensuring that unexpected events or losses do not jeopardize its financial stability. For instance, property insurance can help cover repair or replacement

costs for damaged assets, while business interruption insurance can provide financial support during a temporary closure.

3. **Employee protection:** Insurance policies, such as workers' compensation insurance, protect your staff by covering medical expenses, lost wages, and disability benefits in the event of work-related injuries or illnesses. This coverage not only supports your employees but also helps your center comply with legal requirements and maintain a safe work environment.

4. **Client trust and confidence:** Having appropriate insurance coverage demonstrates your center's commitment to providing high-quality care and maintaining professional standards. This can help instill trust and confidence in your clients, their families, and the broader community, ultimately contributing to the center's overall success and reputation.

5. **Regulatory compliance:** State licensing agencies and local authorities often require specific types and levels of insurance coverage for mental health and addiction treatment centers. Obtaining the necessary coverage ensures your center's compliance with these requirements, preventing potential fines or licensing issues.

6. **Risk management:** Insurance coverage is a key component of effective risk management for your center, helping to mitigate potential risks and minimize their financial impact. By identifying potential threats and securing appropriate coverage,

you can better protect your center from unexpected challenges and focus on providing high-quality care to your clients.

By securing appropriate insurance coverage, you can safeguard your intensive outpatient treatment center's assets, protect its reputation, ensure its financial stability, and promote a safe and supportive environment for both clients and staff. The following insurance coverage should be considered:

a. General Liability Insurance:

General liability insurance is a fundamental type of coverage that protects your intensive outpatient treatment center against claims arising from bodily injury, property damage, and personal injury that occur on your premises or as a result of your center's operations. Some key aspects of general liability insurance include:

b. Premises liability:

Covers injuries or damages sustained by clients, visitors, or third parties while on your center's property, such as slips and falls.

c. Operations liability:

Covers injuries or damages that may occur during the course of providing services, such as during off-site therapy sessions or community outreach events.

d. Personal and advertising injury:

Protects your center against claims related to libel, slander, copyright infringement, or invasion of privacy arising from your advertising or promotional materials.

e. Professional Liability Insurance (Malpractice Insurance):

Professional liability insurance, also known as malpractice insurance, protects your center and its staff from claims related to errors, omissions, or negligence in the provision of professional services. Key components of professional liability insurance include:

i. Coverage for therapists and clinicians: Protects licensed mental health professionals and addiction counselors from claims arising from the therapeutic process, such as misdiagnosis, improper treatment, or breaches of confidentiality.

ii. Coverage for administrative staff: Covers claims related to clerical errors or omissions, such as incorrect billing, scheduling mistakes, or failure to obtain necessary client authorizations.

f. Legal defense and settlement costs:

Provides financial resources to cover legal defense fees, settlement costs, and potential damage awards in the event of a professional liability lawsuit.

g. Workers' Compensation Insurance:

Workers' compensation insurance is a legally required type of coverage that protects your employees in the event of work-related injuries or illnesses. Key aspects of workers' compensation insurance include:

h. Medical expenses:

Covers the cost of medical treatment, hospitalization, and medications required for work-related injuries or illnesses.

i. Lost wages:

Provides financial compensation for employees who are unable to work due to a work-related injury or illness, ensuring they maintain a steady income during their recovery period.

j. Disability benefits:

Offers financial support for employees who suffer a temporary or permanent disability as a result of a work-related injury or illness.

k. Death benefits:

Provides financial assistance to the family or dependents of an employee who dies as a result of a work-related incident.

l. Property Insurance:

Property insurance is an essential type of coverage that protects your center's physical assets, such as buildings, furnishings, and equipment, in the event of damage or loss due to fire, theft, or natural disasters. Key components of property insurance include.

m. Building coverage:

Protects the structure of your center's facility, including any attached fixtures or permanent improvements, in the event of damage or destruction.

n. Contents coverage:

This covers the cost of replacing or repairing your center's furniture, equipment, and other personal property in the event of damage or loss.

o. Business income coverage:

Provides financial assistance to help cover lost revenue and ongoing expenses during the period required to repair or replace damaged property, ensuring your center can maintain its financial obligations during a disruption.

p. Extra expense coverage:

Covers additional costs incurred to continue operations during the repair or replacement process, such as temporary relocation expenses or the cost of renting replacement equipment.

Chapter 3

Medical and Clinical Oversight

Medical and clinical oversight is a crucial aspect of operating a successful intensive outpatient treatment center for mental illness, drug, and alcohol treatment. Ensuring proper medical and clinical oversight is essential for several reasons:

1. Quality of care:

Effective medical and clinical oversight helps ensure that your center provides high-quality care that meets established standards and best practices. This includes implementing evidence-based treatment modalities, providing appropriate supervision of staff, and regularly reviewing treatment outcomes to identify areas for improvement.

Medical and clinical oversight is a critical component of any mental health and addiction treatment center. It ensures that the center provides the highest quality of care and adheres to established standards and best practices. To achieve effective medical and clinical oversight, the center must first identify evidence-based treatment modalities and establish treatment protocols that align with those best practices. This includes ensuring that the center's staff is adequately trained and equipped to implement these protocols.

Another critical element of effective medical and clinical oversight is providing appropriate supervision of staff. The center's clinical director or medical director must ensure that all staff members are adequately trained, qualified, and credentialed to provide the services they offer. They must also monitor staff performance and provide feedback and support as needed to ensure that staff members meet established performance standards.

Regularly reviewing treatment outcomes is also essential to effective medical and clinical oversight. This involves tracking and analyzing client data, including treatment completion rates, improvement in mental health and addiction symptoms, and client satisfaction. By reviewing this data regularly, the center can identify areas for improvement and make data-driven decisions about service improvements.

2. Client safety:

The safety and well-being of your clients is of paramount importance. Proper medical and clinical oversight helps prevent potential harm or adverse events by ensuring that clients receive appropriate treatment, medication management, and monitoring based on their specific needs and diagnoses.

Medical and clinical oversight is essential to ensure the safety and well-being of clients in a treatment center. It involves a comprehensive evaluation of each client's physical and mental health to determine the appropriate course of treatment. This includes medication management, ongoing monitoring of physical and mental health, and regular communication with clients' primary care physicians and other healthcare providers.

Effective oversight also involves the implementation of evidence-based treatment modalities, such as cognitive-behavioral therapy, dialectical behavior therapy, and trauma-focused therapy. These therapies are tailored to each client's specific needs and diagnoses and are regularly monitored to ensure their effectiveness.

Supervision of staff is another critical component of effective medical and clinical oversight. Supervisors should ensure that staff members are properly trained and follow established protocols and procedures. Regular supervision and training can help identify areas for improvement and ensure that staff members provide high-quality care that meets established standards.

3. Regulatory compliance:

State licensing agencies and accreditation organizations often require stringent medical and clinical oversight as part of their compliance standards. Adhering to these requirements helps maintain your center's license and accreditation, and demonstrates a commitment to providing safe, effective care.

State licensing agencies and accreditation organizations have specific requirements for medical and clinical oversight to ensure that treatment centers meet high standards of care. These requirements may include having a licensed physician or psychiatrist on staff to oversee medication management, providing appropriate supervision of licensed and non-licensed staff, and implementing evidence-based treatment modalities.

Adhering to these standards helps ensure that your center provides high-quality care and meets regulatory compliance requirements. By providing appropriate medical and clinical oversight, your center can reduce the risk of harm to clients and improve treatment outcomes. Additionally, demonstrating compliance with these standards can enhance your center's reputation and credibility among clients, staff, and other stakeholders.

4. Staff development and support:

Medical and clinical oversight involves providing guidance, supervision, and ongoing training to your center's clinical staff. This not only ensures that staff members maintain their professional competencies but also creates a supportive work environment that encourages collaboration and continuous improvement.

Medical and clinical oversight provides a framework for ensuring that clinical staff members work together to provide high-quality, evidence-based care that aligns with the center's mission and goals. This includes establishing clinical policies and procedures, developing treatment plans and protocols, and monitoring client progress and outcomes.

Effective clinical oversight requires strong leadership, clear communication, and ongoing training and development for clinical staff members. The clinical oversight team should be comprised of experienced and qualified individuals who possess the necessary expertise to provide guidance and support to staff members.

The clinical oversight team should also stay up-to-date on the latest research and best practices in mental health and addiction treatment, and regularly review and update the center's clinical policies and procedures accordingly.

In addition to providing guidance and supervision, the clinical oversight team should also be responsible for monitoring the quality of care provided by the center. This includes conducting regular audits of clinical documentation, monitoring medication management practices, and ensuring that all staff members are adhering to established clinical protocols.

Overall, effective medical and clinical oversight is essential to ensuring that your center provides safe, effective, and high-quality care to your clients. By establishing clear policies and procedures, providing ongoing training and development for clinical staff, and monitoring the quality of care provided, your center can create a culture of excellence that supports positive client outcomes and fosters professional growth and development for staff members.

5. Risk management:

Proper medical and clinical oversight helps to mitigate potential risks associated with client care, such as medication errors, misdiagnoses, or inappropriate treatment plans. By closely monitoring clinical processes and outcomes, your center can identify and address potential issues before they escalate, minimizing the risk of harm and potential liability.

Proper medical and clinical oversight provides an important layer of protection for both clients and the center. By closely monitoring clinical processes and outcomes, potential risks associated with client care can be mitigated, such as medication errors, misdiagnoses, or inappropriate treatment plans. This helps to ensure that clients receive safe and effective care and reduces the risk of adverse events. Additionally, proper medical and clinical oversight can help protect the center from potential liability by identifying and addressing potential issues before they escalate. Overall, effective medical and clinical oversight is critical to providing high-quality care that meets established standards and best practices.

6. Reputation and credibility:

Demonstrating strong medical and clinical oversight can enhance your center's reputation and credibility in the eyes of clients, referral sources, and the wider community. This, in turn, can help to attract new clients and foster trust in your center's ability to provide effective, high-quality care.

Having a reputation for providing high-quality care is essential for any healthcare organization, including mental health and addiction treatment centers. By implementing effective medical and clinical oversight, your center can demonstrate its commitment to providing safe and evidence-based care, which can build trust and loyalty among clients and referral sources.

This can lead to increased referrals, positive word-of-mouth, and a stronger reputation within the community. Additionally, having a strong reputation can help your center stand out in a crowded marketplace, attracting new clients and helping to ensure long-term sustainability.

7. Coordination of care:

Effective medical and clinical oversight involves coordinating care between various members of the treatment team, such as therapists, psychiatrists, nurses, and case managers. This collaboration ensures that clients receive comprehensive, integrated care that addresses their unique needs and promotes lasting recovery.

Coordination between members of the treatment team is essential to ensure that clients receive the best possible care. Effective medical and clinical oversight involves ensuring that each member of the treatment team understands their role and responsibilities and that there is clear communication and collaboration among team members. This coordination helps to prevent errors and omissions in care and ensures that clients receive consistent, evidence-based treatment throughout their recovery journey.

Medical and clinical oversight may also involve regular team meetings to discuss clients' progress and treatment plans, as well as ongoing training and education for staff members. By maintaining a culture of collaboration and ongoing learning, your center can promote high-quality, effective care and stay up-to-date on the latest best practices and treatment approaches in the field.

8. Outcome measurement and improvement:

Medical and clinical oversight includes tracking and evaluating treatment outcomes, such as client satisfaction, symptom reduction, and improvements in functioning. This data-driven approach allows your center to identify areas for improvement, adjust treatment protocols, and demonstrate the effectiveness of its programs to clients, stakeholders, and regulatory agencies.

By regularly tracking and evaluating treatment outcomes, medical and clinical oversight can help identify areas where clients are not meeting their treatment goals and provide guidance on the most effective interventions to achieve positive outcomes. This data-driven approach can help your center adjust treatment plans and protocols, as well as provide evidence-based results to clients and stakeholders. It also allows your center to continuously improve and innovate its treatment programs, ensuring that they remain up-to-date with the latest research and best practices. Ultimately, effective medical and clinical oversight can help your center provide the highest quality of care and achieve positive outcomes for clients.

By prioritizing medical and clinical oversight, your intensive outpatient treatment center can provide safe, high-quality care to its clients while maintaining regulatory compliance and fostering a supportive, collaborative work environment for its staff.

To ensure the highest quality of care, your center should have:

a. Medical Director:

A medical director is a vital part of an intensive outpatient treatment center's leadership team, responsible for overseeing all medical aspects of the facility's services. The medical director ensures that the center provides safe, effective, and evidence-based care to its clients. Key responsibilities of a medical director include:

1. Developing and implementing medical policies and protocols: The medical director establishes guidelines and procedures related to client assessment, treatment planning, medication management, and emergency response.

2. Coordinating with clinical staff: The medical director collaborates with therapists, counselors, and other mental health professionals to provide integrated care and ensure that clients receive appropriate medical interventions.

3. Overseeing medication management: The medical director supervises the prescription, administration, and monitoring of medications, ensuring that clients receive appropriate pharmacological treatment based on their specific needs and diagnoses.

4. Ensuring regulatory compliance: The medical director ensures that the center meets all applicable medical standards and regulations set forth by licensing agencies and accreditation

organizations.

5. Providing staff training and support: The medical director may provide ongoing education and training to clinical staff, ensuring they stay current with medical advancements and best practices in their fields.

b. Clinical Supervisors:

Clinical supervisors play a crucial role in ensuring the quality and effectiveness of an intensive outpatient treatment center's therapeutic services. They provide guidance, support, and oversight to therapists and other clinical staff members. Key responsibilities of clinical supervisors include:

1. **Supervising clinical staff:** Clinical supervisors provide regular supervision to therapists and other clinical staff, offering guidance on treatment planning, therapeutic interventions, and case management.

2. **Ensuring quality of care:** Clinical supervisors monitor the quality of therapeutic services by regularly reviewing client progress, treatment plans, and clinical documentation to ensure adherence to best practices and established standards.

3. **Supporting staff development:** Clinical supervisors provide ongoing training, feedback, and mentorship to help therapists improve their clinical skills and maintain professional competencies.

4. **Coordinating care:** Clinical supervisors collaborate with the multidisciplinary team to ensure that clients receive comprehensive, integrated care that addresses their unique needs.

5. **Managing client issues and concerns:** Clinical supervisors may address any concerns or issues that arise during therapy, such as ethical dilemmas, therapeutic boundaries, or crisis intervention.

c. A multidisciplinary team of professionals:

A multidisciplinary team of professionals is essential for providing comprehensive, integrated care to clients in an intensive outpatient treatment center. This diverse team of experts works collaboratively to address the various needs and challenges faced by clients. The multidisciplinary team typically includes:

1. **Psychiatrists:** Medical doctors specializing in the diagnosis and treatment of mental health disorders. Psychiatrists can prescribe medications, provide psychotherapy, and manage complex cases that may require additional medical intervention.

2. **Psychologists:** Mental health professionals who provide psychological assessments, diagnosis, and evidence-based therapies, such as cognitive-behavioral therapy or psychodynamic therapy.

3. **Therapists:** Licensed mental health professionals, such as licensed clinical social workers, licensed professional counselors, or marriage and family therapists, who provide individual, group, and family therapy to clients.

4. **Social workers:** Professionals who assist clients with practical needs and challenges, such as housing, employment, and accessing community resources. Social workers may also provide case management services and help clients navigate complex systems.

5. **Addiction counselors:** Certified professionals who specialize in the treatment of substance use disorders. Addiction counselors provide counseling, support, and education to clients and their families, helping them develop coping strategies and relapse prevention.

Chapter 4

Policies and Procedures Manuals

These manuals should cover all aspects of your center's operations, ensuring a comprehensive and efficient framework for providing care. Key components must include:

a. Admission and discharge procedures:

Admission procedures should outline the process for assessing and admitting new clients, including eligibility criteria, intake assessments, and the development of individualized treatment plans. Discharge procedures should define criteria for successful program completion, guidelines for aftercare planning, and the process for transitioning clients to less intensive levels of care or other community resources.

b. Emergency preparedness and response plans:

These plans should detail how the center will respond to various emergencies, such as natural disasters, fires, or medical emergencies. This includes guidelines for staff training, communication protocols, evacuation procedures, and coordination with external agencies. Regular drills and reviews should be conducted to ensure staff preparedness and the effectiveness of the plan.

c. Medication management protocols:

These protocols should outline the proper storage, administration, and documentation of medications, as well as staff responsibilities and training requirements. Additionally, protocols should cover medication reconciliation, error prevention, and the management of side effects, adverse reactions, or medication misuse. Compliance with relevant regulations and best practices should be emphasized.

d. Confidentiality and privacy policies:

These policies should ensure compliance with all applicable privacy laws and regulations, including HIPAA and 42 CFR Part 2. Guidelines should be provided for secure storage and transmission of client information, as well as protocols for addressing potential breaches of confidentiality. Staff should be trained on their responsibilities to protect client privacy and the consequences of violating these policies.

e. Staff and client grievance procedures:

Grievance procedures should offer clear processes for staff and clients to express concerns or complaints, as well as steps for investigation, response, and follow-up. These procedures should emphasize the importance of addressing grievances in a timely, fair, and transparent manner, to resolve issues and maintain a positive, supportive environment for all parties involved.

Policies and procedures manuals are essential tools for the effective operation of an intensive outpatient treatment center. These comprehensive documents serve as guidelines for staff and help ensure consistency, compliance, and quality of care. Developing thorough policies and procedures manuals is vital for several reasons:

1. **Standardization of care:** Policies and procedures manuals establish consistent standards and expectations for all aspects of the center's operation, from client assessments and treatment planning to staff supervision and documentation. This standardization ensures that all clients receive equitable, high-quality care, regardless of the specific staff members involved in their treatment.

2. **Regulatory compliance:** Comprehensive policies and procedures manuals help ensure that your center complies with all applicable state, local, and federal regulations, as well as accreditation requirements. By clearly outlining the center's processes and expectations, these manuals provide staff with the information they need to maintain compliance in their daily work.

3. **Staff training and development:** Policies and procedures manuals serve as valuable resources for staff training and ongoing education. New staff members can reference these manuals to familiarize themselves with the center's operations and expectations while existing staff can consult them to stay current with best practices and evolving standards.

4. **Risk management:** Well-developed policies and procedure manuals help mitigate potential risks by providing clear guidelines for addressing challenging situations, such as client crises, medical emergencies, or ethical dilemmas. By following these established protocols, staff can respond effectively and appropriately, minimizing the potential for harm or liability.

5. **Quality assurance and improvement:** Regularly reviewing and updating policies and procedures manuals ensures that your center's practices remain aligned with current best practices and evidence-based treatment approaches. This ongoing process of quality assurance and improvement helps to optimize client outcomes and maintain the center's reputation for excellence.

Key components of policies and procedures manuals may include:

1. **Admission and intake procedures:** Guidelines for client assessments, diagnostic criteria, and treatment planning, as well as procedures for obtaining informed consent and maintaining client confidentiality.

2. **Treatment protocols:** Detailed descriptions of the center's therapeutic modalities, such as individual, group, and family therapy, as well as evidence-based interventions for specific diagnoses or populations.

3. **Medication management:** Policies and procedures related to the prescription, administration, and monitoring of medications, as well as guidelines for addressing medication-related concerns or

emergencies.

4. **Staff supervision and training:** Expectations for staff supervision, professional development, and performance evaluations, as well as guidelines for addressing staff concerns or conflicts.

5. **Client rights and responsibilities:** Information on clients' rights to privacy, dignity, and respectful treatment, as well as their responsibilities in the therapeutic process.

6. **Crisis intervention and emergency response:** Protocols for managing client crises, medical emergencies, or incidents of violence, including guidelines for involving external support services or emergency responders when necessary.

7. **Documentation and record keeping:** Standards for maintaining accurate, timely, and confidential client records, as well as procedures for releasing information or coordinating care with external providers.

8. **Discharge and aftercare planning:** Guidelines for determining when clients are ready for discharge, as well as processes for developing individualized aftercare plans to support clients in their ongoing recovery. This may include referrals to community resources, support groups, or ongoing outpatient therapy services.

9. **Client engagement and retention strategies:** Policies and procedures to maximize client engagement, promote treatment

adherence, and address issues related to attendance, participation, or dropout. These strategies may include regular progress reviews, motivational interventions, or flexible scheduling options.

10. **Cultural competence and diversity:** Guidelines for ensuring that the center's staff and services are culturally sensitive, inclusive, and respectful of clients' diverse backgrounds, beliefs, and experiences. This may involve staff training in cultural competence, as well as adaptations to treatment approaches or materials to better serve diverse populations.

11. **Confidentiality and HIPAA compliance:** Policies and procedures to protect client's privacy and ensure compliance with the Health Insurance Portability and Accountability Act (HIPAA) and other applicable privacy regulations. This may include guidelines for secure storage and transmission of client information, as well as protocols for addressing potential breaches of confidentiality.

12. **Billing and financial policies:** Guidelines for client billing, insurance verification, and collection procedures, as well as policies related to financial assistance, sliding-scale fees, or payment plans. This section may also address the center's financial management, budgeting, and auditing processes.

13. **Health and safety:** Policies and procedures to ensure a safe and healthy environment for clients and staff, including infection control protocols, maintenance of a clean facility, and guidelines

for addressing potential hazards or emergencies, such as natural disasters or power outages.

14. **Grievance and complaint resolution:** A clear process for clients, family members, or staff to express concerns or grievances and seek resolution, including steps for investigation, response, and follow-up, as well as any relevant reporting requirements.

15. **Performance measurement and evaluation:** Processes for regularly assessing the center's performance and outcomes, including client satisfaction surveys, outcome measurement tools, and quality improvement initiatives. This section may also address the center's commitment to continuous improvement and ongoing evaluation of its programs and services.

16. **Ethical considerations:** Policies and procedures that outline the ethical principles and standards governing the center's operations and staff behavior, including guidelines for addressing ethical dilemmas, maintaining professional boundaries, and avoiding conflicts of interest.

17. **Outreach and community engagement:** Strategies for promoting the center's services, building relationships with referral sources, and collaborating with community organizations to improve access to care and support clients' ongoing recovery. This may include marketing efforts, public education initiatives, or partnerships with local schools, hospitals, or social service agencies.

18. **Technology and electronic health records:** Policies and procedures for using technology in the delivery of care, including electronic health record (EHR) systems, telehealth services, and digital communication tools. This section may also address issues related to data security, privacy, and compliance with relevant regulations.

19. **Substance use policies:** Guidelines for managing substance use and related issues among clients and staff, including policies related to drug testing, medication-assisted treatment, and addressing relapse or substance use during the course of treatment.

20. **Accessibility and accommodation:** Policies and procedures to ensure that the center's facilities and services are accessible to clients with disabilities, as well as guidelines for providing reasonable accommodations as required under the Americans with Disabilities Act (ADA) and other applicable laws.

21. **Incident reporting and response:** Procedures for documenting and responding to incidents or unusual occurrences involving clients or staff, including guidelines for internal investigation, reporting to relevant authorities, and implementing corrective actions to prevent future incidents.

22. **Staff recruitment, hiring, and retention:** Policies and procedures for recruiting, hiring, and retaining qualified staff, including guidelines for background checks, reference verification, and ongoing professional development. This section

may also address strategies for promoting staff satisfaction, teamwork, and engagement.

23. **Facility maintenance and management:** Guidelines for maintaining a clean, safe, and functional facility, including procedures for regular inspections, repairs, and preventive maintenance, as well as protocols for addressing any issues related to facility safety, accessibility, or compliance.

24. **Client and family involvement:** Strategies for involving clients and their families in the treatment process, including guidelines for family therapy, psycho-education, and support services, as well as opportunities for clients and families to provide input on the center's policies, programs, and services.

25. **Volunteer and intern management:** Policies and procedures for recruiting, training, and supervising volunteers and interns, including guidelines for background checks, role assignments, and evaluation processes. This section may also address strategies for creating a positive learning environment and fostering professional growth among volunteers and interns.

26. **Clinical documentation and record-keeping:** Guidelines for the consistent and accurate documentation of clinical services, including progress notes, treatment plans, and discharge summaries. This section should also address the required elements for documentation, timeframes for completion, and processes for review and audit.

27. **Client screening and eligibility criteria:** Policies and

procedures for determining client eligibility for the center's programs and services, including guidelines for assessing the severity of a client's condition, their need for intensive outpatient treatment, and any contraindications or exclusion criteria.

28. **Program evaluation and research:** Processes for evaluating the effectiveness of the center's programs and services, including the use of data-driven decision-making, outcomes measurement, and evidence-based practices. This section may also address the center's commitment to ongoing research and innovation, as well as any collaborations with academic or research institutions.

29. **Emergency preparedness and response:** Guidelines for preparing for and responding to emergencies, such as natural disasters, public health crises, or critical incidents, including plans for staff training, communication, and coordination with external agencies and partners.

30. **Telehealth and remote services:** Policies and procedures for providing telehealth and remote services, including guidelines for technology use, client privacy, and clinical practice standards. This section may also address strategies for ensuring equitable access to remote services and addressing barriers related to technology or digital literacy.

31. **Client satisfaction and feedback:** Processes for collecting and addressing client feedback and satisfaction, including the use of surveys, focus groups, or other methods for gathering input. This section should also outline procedures for reviewing and

responding to feedback, as well as incorporating client perspectives into program improvement efforts.

32. **Continuity of care and care coordination:** Policies and procedures for ensuring seamless transitions between levels of care and providers, including guidelines for coordinating with external providers, sharing client information, and supporting clients during transitions in their treatment journey.

33. **Infection control and hygiene:** Policies and procedures for maintaining a clean and sanitary environment, including guidelines for infection prevention, hand hygiene, and the use of personal protective equipment (PPE). This section should also address procedures for managing communicable diseases and outbreaks, as well as staff training in infection control practices.

34. **Medication storage and disposal:** Guidelines for the proper storage, handling, and disposal of medications, including procedures for managing expired medications, controlled substances, and medication waste. This section should also address staff training and responsibilities related to medication management.

35. **Confidentiality and information sharing:** Policies and procedures for protecting client confidentiality and privacy, including guidelines for sharing client information within the treatment team, with external providers, or with family members. This section should also address compliance with relevant

privacy laws and regulations, such as HIPAA and the 42 CFR Part 2 regulations.

36. **Incident management and critical event debriefing:** Guidelines for managing incidents involving clients or staff, including protocols for documentation, investigation, and follow-up, as well as procedures for conducting critical event debriefings and implementing corrective actions to prevent future incidents.

37. **Quality management and continuous improvement:** Processes for monitoring and improving the quality of the center's programs and services, including the use of performance indicators, quality audits, and feedback mechanisms. This section should also address the center's commitment to evidence-based practices, innovation, and continuous learning.

38. **Nutrition and dietary support:** Policies and procedures for providing clients with appropriate nutrition and dietary support, including guidelines for meal planning, special dietary accommodations, and education on healthy eating habits.

39. **Client rights and grievance procedures:** Guidelines for informing clients of their rights and responsibilities, as well as processes for addressing client grievances, complaints, or concerns in a timely and respectful manner.

40. **Staff wellness and self-care:** Policies and procedures for promoting staff wellness and self-care, including guidelines for managing stress, burnout, and compassion fatigue, as well as resources and support for staff wellbeing.

41. **Substance use testing and monitoring:** Guidelines for conducting substance use testing and monitoring among clients, including protocols for random drug testing, managing positive test results, and addressing relapse or ongoing substance use concerns.

42. **Marketing and community relations:** Policies and procedures for promoting the center's programs and services, including guidelines for marketing materials, media relations, and community outreach efforts.

43. **Facility security and safety:** Guidelines for maintaining a safe and secure environment for clients, staff, and visitors, including procedures for managing access control, security systems, and emergency response.

44. **Crisis intervention and suicide prevention:** Policies and procedures for identifying and responding to clients in crisis, including guidelines for suicide risk assessment, safety planning, and referral to appropriate levels of care.

45. **Staff code of conduct and professional ethics:** Guidelines for staff behavior, professional boundaries, and ethical conduct, including procedures for addressing violations of the code of conduct and disciplinary actions.

46. **Environmental sustainability and resource management:** Policies and procedures for promoting environmental sustainability and responsible resource management, including guidelines for waste reduction, energy conservation, and

environmentally friendly practices.

Chapter 5

Training Manuals and Educational Material

Developing comprehensive training manuals and educational materials is essential for ensuring staff are well-equipped to provide effective care and clients have the resources they need to succeed. Some key topics to cover include:

a. Evidence-based treatment approaches:

Training manuals should provide detailed information on evidence-based treatment approaches for mental health and substance use disorders, including cognitive-behavioral therapy (CBT), dialectical behavior therapy (DBT), motivational interviewing (MI), and trauma-informed care. Staff should be trained to understand the theoretical underpinnings, clinical techniques, and appropriate applications of these approaches, as well as how to tailor them to meet the unique needs of individual clients. Ongoing training and supervision should be provided to support staff in refining their skills and staying up-to-date with the latest research and best practices.

b. Crisis intervention techniques:

Educational materials should cover various crisis intervention techniques, including de-escalation strategies, suicide risk assessment, and safety planning. Staff should be trained to recognize the signs of a potential crisis, respond effectively to clients in distress, and implement appropriate interventions to support clients' safety and well-being. Regular refresher trainings and opportunities for skill practice can help ensure staff are prepared to manage crises with confidence and competence.

c. Cultural competency:

Training manuals should address the importance of cultural competency in providing effective, client-centered care. This includes understanding the impact of culture on mental health, substance use, and help-seeking behaviors, as well as the unique needs and experiences of diverse client populations. Staff should be trained to recognize and address their own biases, develop cultural humility, and adapt their clinical approaches to be more inclusive and responsive to clients' cultural backgrounds. Ongoing training, reflection, and feedback can support staff in continuously improving their cultural competency.

d. Relapse prevention strategies:

Educational materials should provide in-depth information on relapse prevention strategies for clients in recovery from mental health and substance use disorders. This includes understanding the factors that contribute to relapse, identifying early warning signs, and developing personalized coping strategies to manage triggers and maintain progress.

Staff should be trained to support clients in developing and implementing relapse prevention plans, as well as addressing setbacks or relapses compassionately and constructively. Client resources may include self-help materials, psychoeducational workshops, or support groups focused on relapse prevention skills and strategies.

By creating comprehensive training manuals and educational materials on these topics, your intensive outpatient treatment center can ensure staff are knowledgeable, skilled, and prepared to deliver high-quality care, while clients are empowered with the tools and resources they need to achieve lasting recovery.

e. Group facilitation skills:

Training manuals should provide staff with guidance on effective group facilitation skills, such as setting group norms, managing group dynamics, encouraging participation, and addressing challenging behaviors. Staff should be trained in various group therapy models and techniques, including psychoeducational, skills development, process-oriented, and support groups. Ongoing supervision and peer feedback can help staff refine their group facilitation skills and adapt to the diverse needs of clients and group settings.

f. Family involvement and support:

Educational materials should address the importance of family involvement and support in the recovery process. This includes understanding the impact of mental health and substance use disorders on family dynamics, as well as the role of family members in providing support and facilitating change. Staff should be trained in family therapy approaches, psychoeducational interventions, and strategies for engaging family members in the treatment process. Client resources may include family support groups, educational workshops, or family therapy sessions.

g. Co-occurring disorders and integrated treatment:

Training manuals should cover the assessment, diagnosis, and treatment of co-occurring mental health and substance use disorders. Staff should be trained in integrated treatment approaches that address both conditions simultaneously and in a coordinated manner. This includes understanding the complex interplay between mental health and substance use, as well as tailoring interventions to address clients' unique needs and treatment goals. Ongoing training and supervision can support staff in developing the specialized skills and knowledge needed to effectively treat clients with co-occurring disorders.

h. Self-care and staff wellness:

Educational materials should emphasize the importance of self-care and staff wellness in maintaining a healthy, effective treatment team. This includes recognizing the signs of burnout, compassion fatigue, and vicarious traumatization, as well as strategies for managing stress and promoting resilience. Staff should be encouraged to engage in regular self-care practices, seek support from colleagues and supervisors, and prioritize their own well-being. Organizational policies and resources that support staff wellness, such as wellness programs, mental health days, or employee assistance programs, can also be highlighted.

By expanding the training manuals and educational materials to cover these additional topics, your intensive outpatient treatment center can further enhance the quality of care provided, support staff development, and empower clients with the knowledge and resources they need for successful recovery.

i. Client assessment and treatment planning:

Training manuals should provide staff with guidance on conducting comprehensive client assessments and developing individualized treatment plans. This includes understanding the importance of a thorough biopsychosocial assessment, as well as using standardized assessment tools and clinical interviews to gather information on clients' mental health, substance use, and related issues.

Staff should be trained in creating treatment plans that are client-centered, strength-based, and focused on measurable goals and objectives. Ongoing assessment and treatment plan review should be emphasized to ensure that clients' progress is monitored, and interventions are adjusted as needed.

j. Clinical documentation and record-keeping:

Educational materials should cover the importance of accurate, timely, and comprehensive clinical documentation and record-keeping. Staff should be trained in the proper documentation of assessment findings, treatment plans, progress notes, and other relevant clinical information, as well as the use of electronic health record systems. Compliance with relevant regulations, privacy laws, and ethical guidelines should be emphasized, along with the importance of documentation for tracking client progress, demonstrating the effectiveness of interventions, and supporting billing and reimbursement processes.

k. Ethics and professional boundaries:

Training manuals should address the importance of maintaining ethical conduct and professional boundaries in the treatment setting. Staff should be trained to recognize and address potential ethical dilemmas, such as dual relationships, conflicts of interest, or confidentiality breaches. Guidelines for maintaining appropriate professional boundaries with clients, colleagues, and community partners should be provided, along with strategies for addressing boundary violations or ethical concerns. Ongoing training, supervision, and peer consultation can support staff in navigating the complex ethical issues that may arise in their work.

l. Telehealth and digital interventions:

Educational materials should cover the use of telehealth and digital interventions in the delivery of mental health and substance use disorder treatment. Staff should be trained in the effective use of telehealth platforms, as well as the unique considerations and challenges associated with providing care remotely. This includes understanding the importance of maintaining privacy and confidentiality in digital settings, as well as adapting clinical approaches for virtual formats. Training materials should also address the use of digital interventions, such as mobile apps, online support groups, or web-based psychoeducational resources, as adjuncts to traditional treatment approaches.

By further expanding the training manuals and educational materials to include these topics, your intensive outpatient treatment center can provide staff with a comprehensive foundation of knowledge and skills, while equipping clients with a wide range of resources and supports to enhance their recovery journey.

M. Client engagement and retention strategies:

Training manuals should provide staff with strategies for effectively engaging and retaining clients in treatment. This includes understanding the factors that contribute to client engagement, such as rapport-building, empathic communication, and client-centered care.

Staff should be trained in motivational enhancement techniques that help clients recognize the importance of treatment and build their commitment to change. Training materials should also address common barriers to treatment retention, such as transportation, childcare, or financial issues, and guide how to address these challenges and support clients in overcoming them.

n. Trauma-informed care:

Educational materials should address the principles and practices of trauma-informed care in the context of mental health and substance use disorder treatment. Staff should be trained to recognize the signs of trauma, understand the impact of traumatic experiences on clients' mental health, and adapt their clinical approaches to be sensitive to clients' trauma histories. This includes creating a safe and supportive treatment environment, building clients' resilience and coping skills, and integrating trauma-focused interventions as appropriate.

o. Supervision and professional development:

Training manuals should cover the importance of clinical supervision and ongoing professional development for staff working in an intensive outpatient treatment center. Staff should be trained in the process of receiving and providing feedback, engaging in reflective practice, and identifying areas for growth and improvement. Guidelines for establishing and maintaining effective supervisory relationships should be provided, as well as strategies for creating a culture of continuous learning and professional growth within the organization.

p. Community collaboration and resource coordination:

Educational materials should emphasize the importance of collaborating with community partners and coordinating resources to support clients' recovery. Staff should be trained in identifying and establishing relationships with relevant community organizations, such as healthcare providers, social service agencies, housing providers, and peer support groups. Guidance should be provided on how to facilitate smooth transitions and coordinate care across multiple service providers, ensuring that clients have access to the full range of resources and supports needed for successful recovery.

By continuing to expand the training manuals and educational materials to address these additional topics, your intensive outpatient treatment center can further support staff in providing high-quality, comprehensive care to clients, while fostering a culture of collaboration, learning, and continuous improvement.

Chapter 6

Classes and Therapy

Offering a diverse range of classes and therapy modalities ensures that your center can meet the unique needs of each client, providing a comprehensive and individualized approach to treatment. Essential components may include but not be limited to:

a. Group therapy:

Group therapy is a vital part of the treatment process, allowing clients to share their experiences, learn from others, and develop essential social skills. Your center should offer various types of group therapy sessions, such as process groups, skills-based groups, and psychoeducational groups. Facilitators should be trained in group dynamics and effective facilitation techniques, ensuring a safe and supportive environment for all participants. Group therapy sessions should be structured to address specific topics or therapeutic approaches, such as coping skills, relapse prevention, and communication strategies.

Group therapy plays a crucial role in the recovery process by fostering connections among clients, facilitating the exchange of experiences and ideas, and promoting the development of social skills. To provide comprehensive and effective group therapy sessions, your center should offer a variety of group formats, including:

1. Process groups:

Process groups focus on the here-and-now interactions among group members, allowing clients to explore their thoughts, feelings, and behaviors in a safe and supportive environment. Facilitators guide the group's discussion, encouraging members to share their experiences, give and receive feedback, and develop insight into their patterns of relating to others. Process groups can address a wide range of topics, such as relationships, self-esteem, and emotional regulation.

2. Skills-based groups:

Skills-based groups are structured sessions that teach clients practical tools and strategies for managing their mental health and substance use issues. Examples of skills-based groups include DBT skills training, which teaches clients techniques for managing emotions, tolerating distress, and improving interpersonal relationships, and CBT-based relapse prevention groups, which help clients identify triggers, develop coping strategies, and create personalized relapse prevention plans.

3. Psychoeducational groups:

Psychoeducational groups provide clients with information and resources related to mental health, substance use, and recovery. These groups can cover topics such as the neurobiology of addiction, the impact of mental health disorders on daily functioning, and effective strategies for managing stress and emotions. By offering psychoeducational groups, your center empowers clients with the knowledge they need to understand their conditions and take an active role in their recovery.

To ensure the effectiveness of group therapy sessions, facilitators should be trained in group dynamics and facilitation techniques. This includes understanding the stages of group development, managing conflict and resistance, promoting cohesion and engagement, and fostering a therapeutic atmosphere that is safe, supportive, and respectful.

Group therapy sessions should be structured to address specific topics or therapeutic approaches, depending on the needs and goals of the clients. For example, a coping skills group might focus on teaching clients strategies for managing stress and anxiety, while a communication strategies group might help clients develop assertiveness and active listening skills. By offering a variety of group therapy sessions tailored to clients' needs, your center can provide comprehensive and effective support throughout the recovery process.

b. Individual therapy:

Individual therapy provides clients with one-on-one attention and support, allowing for personalized treatment tailored to their unique needs and goals. Your center should employ qualified therapists trained in evidence-based therapeutic approaches, such as cognitive-behavioral therapy (CBT), dialectical behavior therapy (DBT), and trauma-informed care.

Regular individual therapy sessions can help clients address specific issues, develop insight, and build coping skills, all while fostering a strong therapeutic relationship.

Individual therapy is an essential component of comprehensive treatment, as it allows clients to receive personalized care and support that addresses their unique needs, strengths, and goals. In an intensive outpatient treatment center, offering individual therapy can greatly enhance clients' overall recovery process. Some key aspects of individual therapy include:

1. **Personalized treatment:** By working one-on-one with a therapist, clients have the opportunity to explore their specific issues, challenges, and goals in depth. This personalized approach enables the therapist to tailor treatment interventions to the client's unique circumstances, ensuring that therapy is relevant, effective, and aligned with their recovery objectives.

2. **Evidence-based approaches:** Your center should employ

therapists who are trained in evidence-based therapeutic approaches, such as cognitive-behavioral therapy (CBT), dialectical behavior therapy (DBT), and trauma-informed care. These approaches have been proven to be effective in treating a wide range of mental health and substance use disorders, and their integration into individual therapy ensures that clients receive the best possible care.

c. Development of insight and self-awareness:

Individual therapy provides clients with the opportunity to explore their thoughts, feelings, and behaviors in a safe and supportive environment. This process of self-exploration can lead to increased insight and self-awareness, helping clients to better understand the factors that contribute to their mental health or substance use issues and empowering them to make lasting changes in their lives.

1. **Building coping skills:** Through individual therapy, clients can learn and practice a variety of coping skills to manage stress, regulate emotions, and navigate challenging situations. The therapist can help clients identify their existing strengths and develop new skills that are relevant to their specific needs, such as problem-solving, communication, or relaxation techniques.

2. **Fostering a strong therapeutic relationship:** A strong therapeutic relationship is a key factor in successful therapy outcomes. Individual therapy allows clients to develop trust and rapport with their therapist, creating a foundation of safety and

support that enables clients to engage fully in the therapeutic process. By prioritizing the therapeutic relationship, your center can ensure that clients feel understood, valued, and empowered to make meaningful changes in their lives.

3. By offering individual therapy as part of your intensive outpatient treatment center's services, you can provide clients with the personalized attention, support, and evidence-based care they need to address their unique challenges and achieve lasting recovery.

d. Psychoeducational classes:

Psychoeducational classes provide clients with valuable information and resources related to mental health, substance use, and recovery. These classes can cover topics such as the neurobiology of addiction, the impact of mental health disorders on daily functioning, and effective strategies for managing stress and emotions. By offering psychoeducational classes, your center empowers clients with the knowledge they need to understand their conditions and take an active role in their recovery.

Psychoeducational classes play a crucial role in the recovery process by equipping clients with essential knowledge and understanding of mental health, substance use, and recovery. Offering these classes as part of your center's services can help clients make informed decisions about their treatment and actively participate in their recovery journey. Key aspects of psychoeducational classes include:

1. **Understanding the neurobiology of addiction:** One of the primary goals of psychoeducational classes is to help clients

understand the neurobiological basis of addiction. By learning about the brain's reward system, the effects of substances on brain chemistry, and the role of genetic and environmental factors in the development of addiction, clients can better comprehend the complexities of their condition and the importance of seeking treatment.

2. **Exploring the impact of mental health disorders on daily functioning:** Psychoeducational classes can also help clients recognize how mental health disorders affect their daily lives, including their relationships, work, and self-esteem. This awareness can motivate clients to engage in treatment and develop strategies to manage their symptoms and improve their overall quality of life.

3. **Learning effective coping strategies:** Psychoeducational classes can teach clients various coping strategies to manage stress, emotions, and challenging situations effectively. These strategies may include mindfulness techniques, cognitive restructuring, problem-solving skills, and communication strategies. By providing clients with practical tools, your center helps them build resilience and supports their long-term recovery.

4. **Enhancing motivation and commitment to recovery:** Psychoeducational classes can also help clients understand the benefits of treatment and the potential consequences of untreated mental health or substance use disorders. This information can enhance clients' motivation to engage in treatment, set recovery goals, and maintain their commitment to change.

5. **Facilitating informed decision-making:** By offering

psychoeducational classes, your center provides clients with the knowledge they need to make informed decisions about their treatment options and recovery plans. This empowers clients to take an active role in their recovery process and fosters a sense of ownership and responsibility for their well-being.

Incorporating psychoeducational classes into your intensive outpatient treatment center's services can significantly enhance the overall treatment experience for clients. By providing them with valuable information and resources related to mental health, substance use, and recovery, you empower clients to understand their conditions, develop effective coping strategies, and actively participate in their recovery journey.

D. Family therapy:

Family therapy can play a crucial role in the recovery process by addressing the impact of mental health and substance use disorders on family dynamics and relationships. Your center should offer family therapy sessions led by therapists trained in family systems approaches and techniques. Family therapy can help clients and their families develop healthy communication patterns, rebuild trust, and create a supportive home environment conducive to lasting recovery.

Family therapy is an essential component of comprehensive treatment, as it addresses the impact of mental health and substance use disorders on the entire family system. Involving family members in the recovery process can lead to improved treatment outcomes and lasting change. Key aspects of family therapy include:

1. **Addressing family dynamics and patterns:** Family therapy helps clients and their families explore and understand the dynamics and patterns that contribute to the development and maintenance of mental health and substance use disorders. By examining these patterns, families can gain insight into how their interactions and behaviors may inadvertently enable or perpetuate the client's issues, and identify areas for change and growth.

2. **Developing healthy communication skills:** One of the primary goals of family therapy is to help clients and their families develop healthy communication skills. This includes learning how to express emotions, needs, and concerns constructively and respectfully, as well as developing active listening skills. Improved communication can help families resolve conflicts, support each other, and create a more harmonious home environment.

3. **Rebuilding trust and strengthening relationships:** Mental health and substance use disorders can strain family relationships and erode trust among family members. Family therapy can help clients and their families work through past hurts, repair damaged relationships, and rebuild trust. By addressing these issues in therapy, families can move forward with a renewed sense of connection and support.

4. **Establishing healthy boundaries:** Family therapy can also help clients and their families establish healthy boundaries. This

includes setting limits on enabling behaviors, clarifying roles and responsibilities, and developing strategies for maintaining personal well-being while supporting the client's recovery. Establishing healthy boundaries can create a more balanced and supportive family system, ultimately benefiting all members.

5. **Creating a supportive home environment:** A supportive home environment is critical for lasting recovery. Family therapy can help clients and their families identify ways to create a home environment that promotes stability, structure, and positive change. This may involve developing routines, establishing clear expectations, and fostering open communication among family members.

By offering family therapy as part of your intensive outpatient treatment center's services, you provide clients and their families with the tools and support they need to address the complex issues related to mental health and substance use disorders. In doing so, you help clients and their families create a strong foundation for lasting recovery and improved family functioning.

e. Support groups:

Support groups provide clients with a safe space to connect with peers who share similar experiences and challenges. Your center should offer various support groups, such as 12-step meetings, relapse prevention groups, and groups focused on specific mental health disorders or substance use issues. Support groups can help clients build a strong network of social support, reduce feelings of isolation, and develop valuable coping skills through shared experiences.

Support groups are an invaluable resource for clients in recovery, offering a sense of community and understanding that can help individuals navigate the challenges associated with mental health and substance use disorders. By providing access to various support groups, your center can enhance clients' overall treatment experience and contribute to their long-term success. Key aspects of support groups include:

1. **Peer connection and shared experiences:** One of the primary benefits of support groups is the opportunity for clients to connect with peers who share similar experiences and challenges. This sense of camaraderie can help clients feel less isolated and provide a safe space for them to discuss their struggles, accomplishments, and concerns without fear of judgment or stigma.

2. **Social support network:** Participating in support groups can help clients build a strong network of social support, which is crucial for maintaining recovery and preventing relapse. Support from peers can offer encouragement, advice, and understanding during difficult times, helping clients stay committed to their recovery goals.

3. **Skill-building and learning opportunities:** Support groups often provide clients with opportunities to learn from the

experiences of others, as well as share their own insights and strategies for coping with mental health or substance use issues. This exchange of ideas and solutions can help clients develop valuable coping skills and increase their confidence in their ability to manage challenges.

4. **Emotional processing and validation:** Support groups provide clients with a safe space to express their emotions, process their experiences, and receive validation from others who have faced similar challenges. This emotional processing can be therapeutic and contribute to clients' overall well-being and recovery progress.

5. **Specialized focus:** Your center should offer a variety of support groups tailored to the specific needs and interests of your clients, such as 12-step meetings, relapse prevention groups, and groups focused on particular mental health disorders or substance use issues. By providing clients with access to specialized support groups, your center can ensure that clients find the resources and connections most relevant to their recovery journey.

Incorporating support groups into your intensive outpatient treatment center's services can significantly enhance clients' overall treatment experience and contribute to their long-term recovery success. By providing clients with access to a supportive community of peers, your center helps them build the social connections, coping skills, and emotional resilience needed to navigate the challenges of mental health and substance use disorders.

f. Transcranial magnetic stimulation (TMS):

TMS is a non-invasive treatment that uses magnetic fields to stimulate specific areas of the brain associated with mood regulation. Your center could offer TMS as an adjunctive treatment for clients with treatment-resistant depression or other mental health disorders. This would require specialized equipment and trained professionals to administer the treatment safely and effectively.

Transcranial magnetic stimulation (TMS) is an innovative and evidence-based treatment option that can be particularly beneficial for clients who have not responded well to traditional therapies or medications. By offering TMS at your center, you can provide clients with an alternative or adjunctive treatment that may help improve their mental health and overall well-being. Key aspects of TMS include:

1. **Targeted brain stimulation:** works by using magnetic fields to stimulate specific areas of the brain associated with mood regulation, such as the prefrontal cortex. This targeted stimulation can help normalize brain activity in these regions, potentially leading to improvements in mood and mental health symptoms.

2. **Non-invasive treatment:** TMS is a non-invasive treatment, meaning it does not require surgery or anesthesia. Clients remain awake and alert during the procedure, which typically

lasts about 30-60 minutes. This non-invasive approach can make TMS an attractive option for clients who are hesitant about more invasive treatments or those who have not found relief from traditional therapies.

3. **Treatment-resistant depression and other mental health disorders:** TMS is effective in treating treatment-resistant depression, meaning clients who have not experienced significant improvement with other treatment options such as medication or psychotherapy. Additionally, TMS is being studied for its potential benefits in treating other mental health disorders, including anxiety, obsessive-compulsive disorder (OCD), and post-traumatic stress disorder (PTSD).

4. **Specialized equipment and trained professionals:** Offering TMS at your center would require specialized equipment, such as a TMS machine, and trained professionals to administer the treatment safely and effectively. This may involve hiring TMS technicians or training existing staff members in TMS protocols and procedures.

5. **Individualized TMS treatment plans:** TMS treatment plans should be tailored to the specific needs and goals of each client. This may involve adjusting the frequency, intensity, or duration of TMS sessions based on the client's response to treatment and their overall progress in therapy.

By incorporating TMS into your intensive outpatient treatment center's services, you can provide clients with an alternative or adjunctive treatment option that has shown promise in improving mental health and well-being. This innovative treatment can be particularly beneficial for clients who have not found relief with traditional therapies, helping them achieve better outcomes and enhancing their overall treatment experience.

g. Quantitative Electroencephalography (qEEG) and Brain Mapping:

qEEG is a diagnostic tool that measures and analyzes brainwave patterns to identify abnormalities or imbalances that may contribute to mental health or substance use disorders. Your center could incorporate qEEG assessments into the treatment process, informing individualized treatment plans and monitoring clients' progress over time. This would require specialized equipment and trained professionals to conduct the assessments and interpret the results.

Quantitative electroencephalography (qEEG) is a cutting-edge diagnostic tool that can offer valuable insights into clients' brain function and inform individualized treatment plans. By incorporating qEEG assessments and brain mapping into your center's services, you can provide clients with a deeper understanding of their mental health and substance use disorders and demonstrate tangible evidence of their progress over time. Key aspects of qEEG and brain mapping include:

1. **Comprehensive brainwave analysis:** qEEG measures and analyzes brainwave patterns, providing a detailed picture of a

client's brain function. This data can help identify abnormalities or imbalances that may contribute to mental health or substance use disorders, such as overactive or underactive brain regions.

2. **Informing individualized treatment plans:** By incorporating qEEG assessments into the treatment process, clinicians can use the findings to inform individualized treatment plans. This may involve adjusting therapeutic approaches or incorporating adjunctive treatments, such as neurofeedback or TMS, to target specific brain imbalances or abnormalities.

3. **Monitoring progress over time:** qEEG assessments can be conducted periodically throughout a client's treatment to monitor their progress and track changes in their brain function. This ongoing evaluation can help clinicians refine treatment plans and provide clients with tangible evidence of their improvement, potentially increasing motivation and engagement in therapy.

4. **Brain mapping as a visual tool:** Brain mapping, a technique that visually represents qEEG data, can be a powerful tool for demonstrating to clients the changes in their brain function over time. By presenting clients with these visual representations, clinicians can show concrete evidence of improvement, potentially reinforcing clients' commitment to their recovery journey and building their confidence in the treatment process.

5. **Specialized equipment and trained professionals:** Incorporating qEEG assessments and brain mapping into your

center's services would require specialized equipment, such as a qEEG system, and trained professionals to conduct the assessments and interpret the results. This may involve hiring qEEG technicians or training existing staff members in qEEG protocols and procedures.

By offering qEEG assessments and brain mapping at your intensive outpatient treatment center, you can provide clients with a deeper understanding of their brain function and its relationship to their mental health and substance use disorders. Furthermore, by demonstrating tangible evidence of their progress, you can help clients stay engaged and committed to their recovery journey, ultimately contributing to better treatment outcomes and long-term success.

h. Hypnotherapy:

Hypnotherapy uses guided relaxation and focused attention to help clients access their subconscious minds and create positive changes in their thoughts, feelings, and behaviors.

Hypnotherapy is a therapeutic technique that utilizes the power of guided relaxation and focused attention to help clients access their subconscious minds and create lasting positive changes in their thoughts, feelings, and behaviors. By offering hypnotherapy at your intensive outpatient treatment center, you can provide clients with an additional modality to support their recovery and address a wide range of issues. Key aspects of hypnotherapy include:

1. **Accessing the subconscious mind:** During hypnotherapy, clients enter a state of deep relaxation and heightened concentration, allowing them to access their subconscious mind. This state enables clients to be more receptive to positive suggestions and helps them uncover and address deep-rooted issues that may be contributing to their mental health or substance use disorders.

2. **Addressing a variety of issues:** Hypnotherapy can be used to address a wide range of issues, such as anxiety, depression, trauma, self-esteem, stress management, and addictive behaviors. By targeting these issues at their core, hypnotherapy can help clients create lasting changes in their thought patterns and behaviors, ultimately supporting their overall recovery process.

3. **Individualized treatment approach:** Hypnotherapy sessions should be tailored to the specific needs and goals of each client. This may involve using personalized suggestions, visualizations, or therapeutic techniques to address the client's unique challenges and support their individual recovery journey.

4. **Trained hypnotherapists:** Offering hypnotherapy at your center requires employing or contracting with trained and certified hypnotherapists who can safely and effectively guide clients through the process. These professionals should have a solid understanding of hypnosis principles, techniques, and ethical considerations, ensuring that clients receive high-quality care.

5. **Integrating with other treatment modalities:** Hypnotherapy

can be integrated with other evidence-based treatment approaches, such as cognitive-behavioral therapy (CBT), dialectical behavior therapy (DBT), and trauma-informed care. This holistic approach can enhance clients' overall treatment experience and support their progress toward lasting recovery.

By incorporating hypnotherapy into your center's services, you can provide clients with an additional therapeutic modality to help them address deep-rooted issues and create positive changes in their thoughts, feelings, and behaviors. This unique approach can be particularly beneficial for clients who have not found relief with traditional therapies, helping them achieve better outcomes and enhancing their overall treatment experience.

i. Equine therapy:

Equine therapy, also known as equine-assisted therapy, is an experiential therapeutic approach that involves interacting with horses to promote emotional, mental, and physical well-being. By incorporating equine therapy into your intensive outpatient treatment center, you can provide clients with a unique and powerful way to address their mental health and substance use disorders. Key aspects of equine therapy include:

1. **Non-verbal communication and trust building:** Horses are highly sensitive to non-verbal cues and emotions, making them excellent partners in therapy. By interacting with horses, clients can develop a better understanding of their non-verbal

communication and enhance their ability to establish trust and build relationships.

2. **Emotional regulation and self-awareness:** Equine therapy can help clients increase their emotional regulation and self-awareness. By observing and interpreting the horses' reactions to their emotions and behaviors, clients can gain insights into their emotional states and develop healthier coping strategies.

3. **Confidence and self-esteem:** Working with horses can be a powerful way for clients to build confidence and self-esteem. As clients learn to communicate effectively with the animals and complete tasks or challenges, they can develop a greater sense of self-efficacy and personal empowerment.

4. **Social skills and teamwork:** Equine therapy often involves group activities and exercises, which can help clients develop essential social skills and learn the importance of teamwork. Through these experiences, clients can enhance their communication, problem-solving, and conflict resolution abilities, all of which are crucial for maintaining healthy relationships and supporting long-term recovery.

5. **Trained equine therapy professionals:** Offering equine therapy at your center requires trained professionals who are knowledgeable in both equine behavior and mental health therapy. These professionals, often referred to as equine-assisted therapists, should have a strong understanding of the principles and techniques involved in equine therapy and be able to create a

safe and supportive environment for both the clients and the horses.

6. **Facilities and resources:** Incorporating equine therapy into your center's services may require additional facilities, such as a stable or riding arena, as well as access to horses and other necessary resources. It's important to ensure that these facilities and resources meet the highest standards of care and safety for both the clients and the animals involved.

By offering equine therapy at your intensive outpatient treatment center, you can provide clients with an innovative and transformative therapeutic experience that addresses their mental health and substance use disorders uniquely. The powerful connection between clients and horses can lead to profound insights and lasting changes, ultimately supporting clients' overall recovery journey and enhancing their treatment outcomes.

Chapter 7

Billing, Credentialing, and Collections

A successful intensive outpatient treatment center requires a strong financial foundation to provide quality services and maintain long-term viability. To achieve this, you must establish efficient billing, credentialing, and collections processes. These essential components help ensure that your center receives timely payments for services rendered and maintains good standing with insurance providers.

Efficient billing and collections processes: Establishing a streamlined billing and collections process is vital for your center's financial health. This process involves accurately documenting services provided, submitting claims to insurance companies, and collecting payments from clients and insurers. Consider the following best practices for billing and collections:

1. **Use specialized software:** Invest in a reliable billing software system designed for behavioral health services. This software can help automate many aspects of billing, reducing errors and improving efficiency.

2. **Train staff:** Ensure that your administrative staff is well-trained in billing procedures, insurance claim submissions, and managing client accounts.

3. **Monitor accounts receivable:** Regularly review your accounts receivable to identify unpaid claims or overdue client payments. Follow up on these accounts promptly to ensure timely payment.

4. **Establish clear payment policies:** Communicate your center's payment policies to clients at the time of admission. This includes information about insurance coverage, co-pays, deductibles, and self-pay rates.

Credentialing with insurance providers:

Credentialing is the process of becoming an approved provider with insurance companies, allowing your center to accept various insurance plans for your services. The credentialing process involves verifying your center's qualifications, licenses, and compliance with industry standards. Consider the following steps to become credentialed:

1. **Research insurance networks:** Identify the major insurance providers in your area and determine their credentialing requirements.

2. **Submit applications:** Complete and submit the necessary applications and documentation to each insurance provider. This may include information about your center's licenses, certifications, and accreditation.

3. **Maintain up-to-date records:** Regularly update your center's information with insurance providers to ensure continued compliance and good standing.

4. **Stay informed:** Keep abreast of changes in insurance

regulations, industry standards, and credentialing requirements to avoid potential issues.

Regular financial audits and reporting: Conducting regular financial audits and reporting is crucial for maintaining your center's financial stability and identifying areas for improvement. This process involves reviewing your center's financial records, ensuring compliance with applicable laws and regulations, and assessing overall financial performance. Consider the following practices for financial audits and reporting:

1. Develop a financial reporting system:

Establish a system for tracking and reporting your center's financial data, such as revenue, expenses, and accounts receivable.

A financial reporting system is an essential tool for monitoring and managing the financial health of your center. It allows you to track your revenue, expenses, and cash flow, and to identify potential issues or areas for improvement. With a well-designed financial reporting system, you can generate timely and accurate financial statements, such as balance sheets and income statements, which provide valuable insights into your center's financial performance.

To develop a financial reporting system, you will need to identify the key financial metrics that are most relevant to your center's operations and goals. This may include metrics such as revenue per client, client acquisition cost, and average length of stay. You will also need to choose appropriate financial software or tools to manage your financial data and generate reports.

Once your financial reporting system is in place, it is important to regularly review and analyze your financial data to identify trends, opportunities, and potential challenges. By using financial data to inform your decision-making, you can make strategic choices that help your center achieve its financial objectives and better serve its clients.

2. Conduct internal audits:

Regularly perform internal audits to identify discrepancies, inefficiencies, or potential fraud. Use the results to improve your financial processes and internal controls.

Regular internal audits are an important part of ensuring the accuracy and integrity of your center's financial data. By reviewing financial records and processes regularly, you can identify potential errors, discrepancies, or areas of inefficiency that may impact your center's bottom line.

Additionally, regular audits can help detect and prevent fraud or other financial misconduct, ensuring that your center operates with transparency and accountability. Once audit results are obtained, they should be used to improve financial processes and internal controls, promoting stronger financial management and sustainability over the long term.

3. Engage external auditors:

Consider hiring an external auditing firm to conduct periodic financial audits. This can provide an unbiased assessment of your center's financial health and ensure compliance with industry standards and regulations.

Hiring an external auditing firm can bring added credibility to your center's financial reporting and provide an objective assessment of your center's financial performance. External auditors can also identify potential fraud, waste, or abuse in financial operations, which can help prevent financial losses or reputational damage. Additionally, external audits can uncover inefficiencies or areas for improvement in financial processes and controls, enabling your center to operate more efficiently and effectively.

4. Monitor financial performance:

Use financial reports to track your center's performance over time and identify trends, areas of concern, or growth opportunities.

Financial reports provide a snapshot of your center's financial health, including revenue, expenses, and cash flow. By analyzing this data over time, you can identify trends and patterns that may indicate areas for improvement or opportunities for growth. For example, if you notice a consistent increase in revenue from a particular service, you may consider expanding that service or investing in marketing to attract more clients. Additionally, financial reports can help you make informed decisions about budgeting, pricing, and staffing, ensuring that your center operates efficiently and sustainably.

By implementing efficient billing, credentialing, and collections processes, your intensive outpatient treatment center can maintain a solid financial foundation, which is crucial for providing quality care and supporting long-term success. Regularly monitoring and evaluating these processes can help you address potential issues, optimize financial performance, and ensure that your center remains compliant with industry standards and regulations.

Chapter 8

Employee Management

Effective employee management is crucial for maintaining a high-quality, dedicated workforce in your intensive outpatient treatment center. By focusing on hiring, training, and supporting your staff, you can create a positive work environment that promotes professional growth and exceptional patient care. Consider the following key aspects of employee management:

1. Hiring qualified staff members:

Recruiting and retaining highly skilled professionals is a critical component of providing high-quality services to clients. Consider implementing the following best practices to attract and retain top talent:

a. Offer competitive compensation packages: Compensation is a key factor in attracting and retaining qualified staff members. Ensure that your center offers competitive salaries, benefits, and opportunities for professional development.

b. Provide a supportive work environment: Creating a

supportive work environment that promotes work-life balance, open communication, and teamwork can help reduce staff turnover and increase job satisfaction.

c. Invest in staff training and development: Providing ongoing training and professional development opportunities can help staff members stay up-to-date on the latest research, trends, and best practices in mental health and addiction treatment.

d. Foster a culture of collaboration and continuous learning: Encourage staff members to share their knowledge and expertise with one another and to collaborate on treatment plans and program development.

e. Recognize and reward staff members for their contributions: Regularly acknowledge and reward staff members who demonstrate exceptional performance or make significant contributions to your center's success. This can include bonuses, promotions, or public recognition.

2. Develop clear job descriptions:

Clearly outline the qualifications, skills, and responsibilities required for each position. Providing a clear and detailed job description for each position can help attract qualified candidates who possess the required skills and experience. The job description should outline the essential functions, required qualifications, and preferred experience for each role.

This information can help potential applicants assess whether they are a good fit for the position and can also help your center streamline the recruitment process by attracting candidates who are well-suited to the role. Additionally, clear job descriptions can help your center avoid potential misunderstandings or conflicts with staff members regarding job expectations and responsibilities.

3. Use multiple recruitment channels:

Advertise job openings on industry-specific job boards, social media, and professional networks to attract a diverse pool of candidates. Expanding on this, advertising job openings on industry-specific job boards such as Psychology Today, Substance Abuse and Mental Health Services Administration (SAMHSA), and National Council for Behavioral Health, can help you reach qualified candidates who are interested in mental health and addiction treatment work.

Utilizing social media platforms like LinkedIn, Twitter, and Facebook can also help you reach a wider audience and potentially attract candidates who may not have been actively searching for a job. Additionally, networking with professional organizations and attending job fairs or career events can provide opportunities to meet potential candidates face-to-face and build relationships with industry professionals.

4. Conduct thorough interviews:

Implement a structured interview process to evaluate candidates' skills, experience, and cultural fit. A structured interview process involves developing a standardized set of questions for each candidate, allowing for a fair and objective evaluation. This can include behavioral-based questions that assess how candidates have handled similar situations in the past, as well as questions that assess their knowledge and skills related to the position.

It's important to ensure that all interviewers are trained on the process and evaluate candidates consistently. This helps to reduce biases and increase the likelihood of selecting the most qualified candidate for the role.

5. Verify credentials:

Verify candidates' licenses, certifications, and educational backgrounds to ensure they meet the requirements for their respective roles. Verifying candidates' licenses, certifications, and educational backgrounds is a critical step in the recruitment process to ensure that they possess the necessary qualifications and meet regulatory requirements for their roles. This verification process may involve checking with state licensing boards, contacting educational institutions, and confirming certification status with relevant credentialing bodies. Conducting these checks can help to prevent potential legal and ethical issues and safeguard the quality of care provided by your center.

6. Offer competitive compensation and benefits:

Attract and retain top talent by offering competitive salaries, benefits, and opportunities for professional development. Offering competitive salaries and benefits is an important aspect of attracting and retaining top talent. Conduct research to understand industry standards for salaries and benefits and aim to offer packages that are in line with those expectations. In addition to financial compensation, consider offering opportunities for professional development, such as continuing education courses, conferences, and leadership training. Providing opportunities for growth and advancement can help motivate staff and increase job satisfaction. Finally, creating a positive work culture that fosters collaboration, open communication, and a healthy work-life balance can also help retain top talent.

Providing ongoing training and support: Invest in your staff's professional growth by offering ongoing training and support. This can help your employees stay current on best practices, enhance their skills, and maintain high standards of care. Consider the following strategies:

1. Offer in-house training:

Organize regular workshops, seminars, and training sessions on relevant topics, such as evidence-based treatment approaches, crisis intervention techniques, and cultural competency. Organizing regular workshops, seminars, and training sessions on relevant topics can help your staff stay up-to-date on the latest research and best practices in the field of mental health and addiction treatment. This not only benefits clients by ensuring they receive the most effective care, but it also helps staff feel supported and valued, leading to greater job satisfaction and retention. Providing ongoing training can also help staff develop new skills and competencies, which can translate into improved client outcomes and enhanced center performance. Additionally, offering professional development opportunities can help your center stand out as a desirable employer and attract top talent in the industry.

2. Encourage external training:

Support staff in attending conferences, workshops, or courses offered by professional organizations or industry experts. Encouraging staff to attend conferences, workshops, or courses offered by professional organizations or industry experts can help them stay up-to-date with the latest trends, research, and best practices in mental health and addiction treatment. It also provides opportunities for networking and professional growth. By supporting staff in continuing education and training, your center can improve the quality of care and attract and retain highly skilled professionals.

3. Implement a mentorship program:

Pair new staff members with experienced professionals who can offer guidance, support, and feedback during their onboarding process. Pairing new staff members with experienced professionals can be an effective way to facilitate their onboarding process. This approach allows new hires to learn from experienced professionals and familiarize themselves with the center's policies, procedures, and culture. This can help to minimize errors, reduce turnover, and improve the quality of care provided to clients.

Experienced professionals can serve as mentors, providing guidance and support to new staff members as they navigate their roles and responsibilities. They can also offer constructive feedback on their performance, identify areas for improvement, and provide opportunities for growth and development.

Pairing new staff members with experienced professionals can also help to build a sense of community and connection within the center. It can foster a culture of learning and collaboration, where staff members feel supported and valued, which can contribute to their job satisfaction and motivation.

4. Promote a culture of continuous learning:

Encourage open communication, collaboration, and knowledge sharing among your team members. Encouraging open communication, collaboration, and knowledge sharing among team members is crucial for creating a supportive and productive work environment.

This can be achieved through regular team meetings, feedback sessions, and brainstorming sessions. Providing opportunities for staff members to share their experiences, ideas, and best practices not only helps to build camaraderie and promote teamwork but also fosters innovation and continuous improvement. Encouraging open communication can also help to identify potential issues or challenges in client care and develop effective solutions as a team.

Establishing performance evaluations: Regular performance evaluations help identify areas of strength and areas for improvement, fostering professional growth and ensuring high-quality patient care. Consider the following best practices for performance evaluations:

1. **Develop clear performance metrics:** Establish objective criteria for evaluating staff performance, such as client outcomes, adherence to treatment protocols, and teamwork.

2. **Conduct regular evaluations:** Schedule performance evaluations at consistent intervals, such as annually or semi-annually, to provide timely feedback and support.

3. **Use a structured feedback process:** Implement a standardized process for providing constructive feedback, including specific examples and recommendations for improvement.

4. **Encourage self-assessment:** Invite staff members to reflect on their performance and set personal goals for improvement.

Implementing clear policies for promotions, terminations, and disciplinary actions:

1. Establishing clear policies for promotions, terminations, and disciplinary actions helps create a fair and transparent work environment. This can contribute to staff satisfaction, motivation, and retention. Consider the following guidelines:

2. Develop clear promotion criteria: Outline the requirements for promotions, such as performance metrics, years of experience, and additional training or certifications.

3. Establish a fair and transparent termination process: Create a standardized process for terminations, including clear documentation of performance issues and opportunities for

improvement.

4. Implement disciplinary procedures: Develop a formal policy for addressing performance or conduct issues, including warnings, performance improvement plans, and potential consequences.

5. Communicate policies clearly: Ensure that all staff members are aware of your center's policies regarding promotions, terminations, and disciplinary actions. By focusing on these aspects of employee management, you can create a strong, dedicated workforce committed to providing exceptional care and support to your clients. Investing in your staff's professional development, providing ongoing feedback and support, and maintaining fair and transparent policies can contribute to a positive work environment and long-term success for your intensive outpatient treatment center.

Fostering a positive work environment: Creating a positive work environment is essential for maintaining staff satisfaction, motivation, and retention. A supportive and inclusive atmosphere can help your employees feel valued, connected, and engaged in their work. Consider the following strategies for fostering a positive work environment:

a. Encourage open communication: Promote a culture of open communication, where employees feel comfortable sharing ideas, concerns, and feedback with their colleagues and supervisors.

b. Recognize and reward achievements: Acknowledge and celebrate the accomplishments of your staff, whether through verbal praise, formal recognition programs, or incentive-based rewards.

c. Offer opportunities for team building: Organize regular team-building activities, such as retreats, workshops, or social events, to strengthen relationships among staff members and foster a sense of camaraderie.

d. Prioritize employee well-being: Implement programs and policies that support employee well-being, such as flexible work hours, mental health resources, and stress management initiatives.

e. Ensure diversity and inclusion: Create an inclusive work environment by promoting diversity and ensuring equal opportunities for all staff members, regardless of their background, gender, race, or other factors.

Implementing effective employee onboarding: A well-structured onboarding process can help new employees feel welcome, supported, and prepared for their roles. This can contribute to job satisfaction, performance, and retention. Consider the following best practices for employee onboarding:

1. **Develop a comprehensive orientation program:** Provide new employees with an overview of your center's mission, values, policies, and procedures, as well as an introduction to their

specific job responsibilities.

2. **Assign a mentor or buddy:** Pair new employees with experienced colleagues who can provide guidance, support, and feedback during their initial weeks on the job.

3. **Offer ongoing training:** Ensure new employees receive appropriate training on evidence-based treatment approaches, crisis intervention techniques, and other relevant topics.

4. **Monitor progress and provide feedback:** Regularly check in with new employees to assess their progress, address any concerns, and provide constructive feedback.

5. **Gather feedback from new employees:** Solicit feedback from new employees about their onboarding experience to identify areas for improvement and make adjustments as needed.

By focusing on these aspects of employee management, your intensive outpatient treatment center can build a dedicated, skilled workforce capable of providing exceptional care to clients. This will contribute to the overall success of your center and help ensure the well-being of your clients and staff alike.

Chapter 9

Marketing and Advertising

You will need to promote your center through various marketing channels, such as:

Building a professional website:

A well-designed and informative website is essential for attracting clients and establishing credibility for your center. Consider the following best practices for building a professional website:

1. Easy navigation:

Ensure your website is easy to navigate, with clearly labeled menus and links to essential pages such as services, staff profiles, and contact information.

Expanding on the statement, having a website that is user-friendly and easy to navigate can enhance the overall experience for clients and visitors to your website. A clear and organized website structure with easy-to-find information can also increase the likelihood of potential clients contacting your center or exploring your services further.

It's important to ensure that the website's content is up-to-date, relevant, and accessible to people with disabilities. Including a blog section or a news page that features regular updates on industry-related news and events can also help establish your center as a reputable and knowledgeable resource in the field. Additionally, incorporating features such as an online scheduling system, a virtual tour of your center, or a chatbot for answering common questions can enhance the user experience and streamline the process of connecting with your center.

2. Engaging content:

Provide engaging and informative content that highlights your center's unique offerings, treatment approaches, and success stories.

To expand, having engaging and informative content on your center's website is essential to attract potential clients, build trust and credibility, and differentiate your center from others in the field. This content can include descriptions of your programs and services, information about your staff and their qualifications, educational resources on mental health and addiction, and success stories from former clients.

By highlighting your center's unique offerings, treatment approaches, and outcomes, you can effectively communicate your value proposition and appeal to the needs and preferences of your target market. Additionally, regularly updating your website with fresh, relevant content can improve your search engine rankings and drive traffic to your site.

3. Search engine optimization (SEO):

Optimize your website for search engines by using relevant keywords, quality content, and proper meta tags. This will help potential clients find your center when searching for treatment options online.

Expanding on the point, search engine optimization (SEO) is a crucial aspect of digital marketing that can help improve the visibility and traffic of your website. By using relevant keywords and phrases in your website's content, you can increase your chances of appearing on the first page of search engine results pages (SERPs) for specific search queries related to your services.

Additionally, creating quality content that is valuable and informative to your target audience can attract more visitors to your website and improve your website's overall SEO. Other factors that can impact your website's search engine ranking include website speed, mobile responsiveness, and user experience, so it's important to ensure that your website is optimized for these factors as well.

4. Mobile-friendly design:

Ensure your website is responsive and accessible on various devices, including smartphones and tablets, as many people use mobile devices to search for information.

Making your website responsive and accessible on various devices, including smartphones and tablets, is important because a significant number of people use mobile devices to access the internet. A responsive website will adapt to different screen sizes and orientations, making it easy to navigate and view on any device. This can improve the user experience and increase the likelihood of potential clients staying on your website and learning more about your center.

Additionally, ensuring that your website is accessible to individuals with disabilities, such as those who are visually impaired or have mobility impairments, can help to expand your potential client base and demonstrate your center's commitment to inclusivity.

5. Clear calls to action:

Include clear calls to action throughout your website, such as contact forms, phone numbers, or email addresses, to encourage potential clients to reach out and learn more about your center.

Calls to action are important prompts that encourage website visitors to take a specific action, such as contacting your center or scheduling an appointment. By strategically placing calls to action throughout your website, you can guide potential clients toward taking the next step in seeking treatment.

For example, you can include a "Contact Us" button on the homepage or a "Schedule a Consultation" form on the services page. Including calls to action in multiple locations can help ensure that visitors see them and are encouraged to take action.

Additionally, it's important to make sure that the calls to action are clear and easy to follow. Use language that communicates the action you want visitors to take and make sure the buttons or forms are prominently displayed and easy to use.

By including effective calls to action on your website, you can increase the likelihood of converting website visitors into potential clients and ultimately, improve your center's success in helping individuals with mental health and addiction issues.

Utilizing social media platforms: Social media platforms, such as Facebook, Instagram, Twitter, and LinkedIn, can help you reach a wider audience and engage with potential clients. To make the most of social media marketing, consider the following strategies:

1. **Share relevant content:** Regularly post informative and engaging content related to mental health, substance use, and recovery. This can include articles, videos, infographics, and personal stories.

2. **Interact with your audience:** Respond to comments and messages promptly, and engage with your followers by asking questions and encouraging discussions.

3. **Use targeted advertising:** Utilize paid advertising options on social media platforms to reach specific demographics or geographic areas.

4. **Promote events and updates:** Share news about upcoming events, staff achievements, or other notable updates related to your center.

5. **Monitor your online reputation:** Keep track of your center's

online reviews and reputation, addressing any negative feedback and showcasing positive testimonials.

Networking with local healthcare providers: Establish relationships with local healthcare providers, such as primary care physicians, psychiatrists, and therapists, who may refer clients to your center. Attend networking events, join professional organizations, and offer educational workshops or presentations to connect with other professionals in your community.

Hosting open houses and community events:

Organize open houses, community workshops, or educational events to raise awareness about your center and the services you provide. These events can help you connect with potential clients, their families, and other professionals in your community. Offer tours of your facility, introduce your staff and provide informative presentations on topics relevant to mental health and addiction treatment.

Content marketing and blogging:

Create and share valuable content related to mental health, addiction treatment, and recovery through a blog on your website. By regularly posting informative articles, you can establish your center as a trusted resource and increase your online visibility. Consider guest blogging opportunities on reputable websites to further expand your reach and credibility.

Public relations and media outreach:

Develop a public relations strategy to promote your center's successes, partnerships, and events in local and national media. Reach out to journalists, bloggers, and influencers in the mental health and addiction treatment space to share your stories and pitch relevant topics. Press coverage can help increase awareness of your center and its services, boosting your reputation and attracting new clients.

Email marketing:

Build a mailing list of potential clients, families, and professional contacts to keep them informed about your center's services, events, and news. Create engaging newsletters and email campaigns to nurture relationships with your audience and encourage them to consider your center for their treatment needs. Be sure to follow best practices for email marketing, such as segmenting your audience, using personalized content, and tracking your results.

Local advertising:

Invest in local advertising through traditional media channels such as print, radio, or television, to reach potential clients in your community. Consider sponsoring local events or partnering with community organizations to increase your visibility and demonstrate your commitment to addressing mental health and addiction issues in your area.

Collaborating with schools and universities:

Partner with local schools and universities to offer educational workshops, presentations, and resources related to mental health and addiction prevention. These collaborations can help you connect with potential clients, their families, and school professionals who may refer students to your center for treatment.

Video marketing:

Leverage the power of video to showcase your center's unique offerings, treatment approaches, and success stories. Create informative and engaging videos for your website, social media platforms, and YouTube channel. Videos can include interviews with staff, testimonials from clients and their families, facility tours, and educational content related to mental health and addiction treatment.

Online webinars and virtual events:

Organize online webinars, workshops, or support groups to reach potential clients who may not be able to attend in-person events. Virtual events can help you connect with a broader audience, provide valuable information, and showcase your center's expertise in mental health and addiction treatment. Promote your virtual events through your website, social media channels, and email marketing campaigns.

Search engine marketing (SEM):

Invest in search engine marketing strategies, such as pay-per-click (PPC) advertising, to increase your center's visibility in search engine results pages. PPC advertising allows you to bid on relevant keywords and target specific demographics, ensuring your ads reach the right audience. Monitor your ad performance and adjust your bidding and targeting strategies as needed to optimize results and maximize your return on investment.

Partnering with other community organizations:

Collaborate with other community organizations, such as nonprofits, support groups, and treatment centers, to increase your center's visibility and reach. By partnering with these organizations, you can share resources, referrals, and co-host events to better serve your clients and their families.

Influencer marketing:

Identify influencers in the mental health and addiction treatment space who can help promote your center and its services. This may include popular bloggers, social media personalities, or experts in the field. Collaborate with influencers to create sponsored content, co-host events, or participate in joint campaigns to reach new audiences and increase your center's visibility.

By continuously exploring new marketing and advertising avenues, you can stay ahead of the competition and ensure your center remains an attractive option for potential clients seeking treatment. Regularly evaluate the effectiveness of your strategies and be prepared to adapt to changing market conditions and emerging trends in the mental health and addiction treatment landscape.

Networking with local healthcare providers:

Building strong relationships with local healthcare providers is essential for increasing referrals and establishing your center as a trusted resource in the community. To network effectively with healthcare providers:

1. Identify potential referral sources, such as primary care physicians, psychiatrists, psychologists, therapists, hospitals, and other treatment centers.

2. Attend professional events, such as conferences, workshops, and seminars, where you can meet and network with healthcare providers in your area.

3. Join local healthcare associations, chambers of commerce, or other professional groups to connect with healthcare providers and stay informed about industry trends and developments.

4. Offer to provide educational presentations or workshops to healthcare providers about your center's services and the benefits of intensive outpatient treatment for mental health and addiction.

5. Maintain regular communication with healthcare providers through email updates, newsletters, or personal visits to their offices. Keep them informed about your center's programs, success stories, and any new services or treatment approaches you may be offering.

6. Consider hosting a regular networking event or open house at your center specifically for healthcare providers. This allows them to tour your facility, meet your staff, and learn more about the services you provide.

Hosting open houses and community events:

Open houses and community events can help raise awareness about your center, showcase your services, and build relationships with potential clients, their families, and local healthcare providers. To host successful events:

1. Plan your event well in advance, giving yourself ample time to promote it and coordinate logistics.

2. Select a date and time that is convenient for your target audience, such as evenings or weekends, when more people may be available to attend.

3. Choose an event format that highlights your center's strengths and services, such as a facility tour, informational presentation, panel discussion, or interactive workshop.

4. Promote your event through various channels, including your website, social media platforms, local media, and email marketing campaigns. Consider creating eye-catching flyers or posters to distribute in your community.

5. Collaborate with local healthcare providers, schools, or community organizations to co-host or sponsor your event. This can help increase your event's visibility and credibility.

6. Provide refreshments, giveaways, or promotional items to encourage attendance and leave a positive impression on attendees.

7. Make sure your center is clean, well-organized, and professionally presented on the day of the event.

8. Have knowledgeable staff members available to answer

questions, provide information, and engage with attendees.

9. Collect contact information from attendees for follow-up communication and future marketing efforts.

By hosting open houses and community events, you can strengthen your center's presence in the community, attract new clients, and establish valuable connections with local healthcare providers and other stakeholders.

Chapter 10

Daily Scheduling and Operations

Daily scheduling and operations are crucial aspects of running a successful intensive outpatient treatment center. A well-organized and efficient schedule ensures clients receive the appropriate level of care and support while maximizing the use of your center's resources. To effectively manage daily scheduling and operations, consider the following steps:

1. **Develop a master schedule:** Create a master schedule that outlines the timing and frequency of all services offered at your center, such as group therapy sessions, individual therapy appointments, psychoeducational classes, and support groups. Ensure that the schedule is designed to provide a balanced mix of therapeutic interventions, educational opportunities, and downtime for clients.

2. **Allocate resources:** Determine the staffing, space, and equipment requirements for each service and allocate the necessary resources accordingly. This may involve scheduling multiple therapists to facilitate group sessions or reserving specific rooms for individual therapy appointments.

3. **Establish a booking system:** Implement a user-friendly booking system that allows clients to schedule appointments for individual therapy, family therapy, or other services. Ensure that the system is accessible to clients and staff members and can be easily updated to reflect changes in availability.

4. **Coordinate staff schedules:** Coordinate the schedules of your clinical staff, administrative staff, and support staff to ensure adequate coverage and smooth daily operations. Consider using scheduling software to manage staff schedules, time-off requests, and shift changes.

5. **Monitor client progress:** Regularly review the progress of each client to ensure they are receiving the appropriate level of care and support. Adjust their individual treatment plans and daily schedules as needed to address any emerging needs or challenges.

6. **Maintain clear communication:** Ensure that all staff members are informed of any changes to the daily schedule or operational procedures. Hold regular staff meetings to discuss client progress, address any concerns, and share important updates.

7. **Implement contingency plans:** Develop contingency plans to address unexpected events, such as staff absences or facility issues, that may disrupt daily operations. Ensure that all staff members are aware of these plans and know how to respond in the event of an emergency.

8. **Evaluate and adjust:** Continuously evaluate the effectiveness of your daily scheduling and operational processes, and be prepared to make adjustments as needed. Solicit feedback from clients and staff members to identify areas for improvement or potential bottlenecks in service delivery. By prioritizing daily scheduling and operations, you can create a structured and supportive environment that promotes recovery and fosters client success. A well-managed schedule ensures that clients receive the appropriate level of care while maximizing the use of your center's resources, ultimately contributing to the overall success of your intensive outpatient treatment program.

9. **Flexibility in scheduling:** Ensure that your daily schedule has some flexibility to accommodate unforeseen circumstances or individual client needs. This may involve having a buffer time between appointments or providing alternative options for clients who cannot attend a scheduled session.

10. **Time management training for staff:** Provide time management training for your staff to help them manage their workload effectively and ensure smooth daily operations. This may include teaching strategies for prioritizing tasks, setting realistic deadlines, and balancing client care with administrative duties.

11. **Streamlining administrative processes:** Review your center's administrative processes regularly and identify opportunities to streamline or automate tasks. This may include using electronic health records, automating appointment reminders, or

integrating billing and scheduling software. Reducing the administrative burden on staff allows them to focus on delivering high-quality care to clients.

12. **Regularly review and update the schedule:** Review the master schedule at regular intervals to ensure that it continues to meet the needs of your clients and staff. This may involve adding new services, adjusting the frequency of existing services, or reallocating resources to accommodate changes in demand.

13. **Client input in scheduling:** Seek feedback from clients about their preferred appointment times, the frequency of sessions, and the types of services they find most beneficial. Incorporate this feedback into the scheduling process to create a client-centered environment that supports their recovery.

14. **Collaboration with external providers:** Collaborate with external providers, such as psychiatrists, primary care physicians, or case managers, to coordinate care and ensure that clients receive the appropriate services and support. This may involve sharing updates on client progress, adjusting treatment plans, or scheduling joint appointments.

15. **Monitor staff workload and well-being:** Monitor the workload and well-being of your staff to ensure they are not overwhelmed or experiencing burnout. Provide opportunities for self-care, professional development, and peer support to help maintain a healthy and motivated workforce.

16. **Client orientation and onboarding:** Develop a thorough

orientation process for new clients, providing them with an overview of the center's services, daily schedule, and expectations. This will help clients feel more comfortable and prepared as they begin their treatment journey.

17. **Implement a tiered service model:** Consider implementing a tiered service model that offers varying levels of care and support based on each client's individual needs. This can help manage the daily schedule more effectively and ensure clients receive the appropriate services at each stage of their recovery.

18. **Utilize technology:** Embrace technology to enhance scheduling and communication, such as using mobile apps for appointment reminders, telehealth services for remote sessions, or digital tools for treatment planning and progress tracking.

19. **Regularly assess facility needs:** Evaluate the physical layout and capacity of your center regularly to ensure it meets the needs of your clients and staff. This may involve rearranging spaces, adding new rooms or equipment, or addressing any maintenance issues that arise.

20. **Create a positive work environment:** Foster a positive work environment that encourages teamwork, open communication, and a shared commitment to client success. This can help improve staff morale and productivity, ultimately contributing to more effective daily operations.

21. **Develop a client-centered scheduling approach:** Adopt a client-centered approach to scheduling that prioritizes the needs

and preferences of clients while balancing the demands of the center. This may involve offering flexible appointment times, accommodating special requests, or adjusting the schedule based on client feedback.

22. **Track key performance indicators (KPIs):** Monitor key performance indicators (KPIs) related to daily scheduling and operations, such as client satisfaction, staff productivity, and resource utilization. Regularly review these metrics to identify areas for improvement and inform data-driven decision-making.

23. **Ongoing staff training and development:** Provide ongoing training and development opportunities for your staff to help them stay current with industry best practices and enhance their skills. This can lead to more effective daily operations and improved client outcomes.

24. **Continuity of care:** Ensure continuity of care for clients by maintaining consistent scheduling and staffing arrangements. This can help build strong therapeutic relationships and promote a sense of stability and predictability for clients.

By focusing on these additional aspects of daily scheduling and operations, you can further enhance the efficiency and effectiveness of your intensive outpatient treatment center. A well-managed center promotes client recovery and staff satisfaction, contributing to the overall success of your program and establishing your facility as a trusted provider in the community.

Conclusion

In conclusion, opening and operating a successful intensive outpatient treatment center for mental illness, drug, and alcohol treatment requires careful planning, attention to detail, and a commitment to providing high-quality care. This guidebook has outlined the essential steps and considerations for establishing your center, from obtaining state licensing and local business permits to implementing comprehensive policies and procedures, securing proper insurance coverage, and offering a diverse array of therapeutic services.

Your center's success will depend on your ability to assemble a dedicated team of professionals, create a supportive and healing environment for clients, and maintain efficient daily operations. Additionally, effective marketing and advertising strategies will help build awareness of your center within the community and attract clients who can benefit from your services.

Remember that the journey to opening and operating a successful intensive outpatient treatment center is an ongoing process. Continuously evaluate and improve your center's operations, stay informed about industry best practices, and adapt your services to meet the changing needs of your clients. By maintaining a strong commitment to excellence and prioritizing the well-being of both clients and staff, you can create a thriving outpatient treatment program that makes a lasting impact on the lives of those you serve.

As your intensive outpatient treatment center continues to grow and evolve, it's essential to remain focused on your mission and the core values that guide your organization. By keeping the well-being of your clients at the forefront of every decision, you can ensure that your center remains a valuable resource for individuals and families in need of support.

To stay ahead in the field, consider the following additional tips for long-term success:

1. **Engage in continuous quality improvement:** Regularly review your center's performance and identify areas for improvement. Seek feedback from clients, staff, and stakeholders to inform your quality improvement efforts and ensure that your center remains responsive to the needs of the community.

2. **Stay informed about industry trends and best practices:** Attend conferences, workshops, and training sessions to stay up to date on the latest developments in mental health and addiction treatment. Networking with other professionals can also provide valuable insights and foster collaboration within the field.

3. **Cultivate partnerships with other organizations:** Collaborate with other treatment centers, healthcare providers, and community organizations to expand your center's referral network and enhance the services available

to clients. These partnerships can also create opportunities for joint initiatives and programs that benefit the broader community.

4. **Invest in staff development and well-being:** Prioritize staff training, professional development, and self-care to promote a healthy work environment and retain skilled professionals. Providing opportunities for growth and advancement can help staff members feel valued and engaged in their work.

5. **Monitor and adapt to changes in regulations and funding:** Stay abreast of changes in state and federal regulations, as well as funding opportunities that can impact your center's operations. Being proactive in adapting to these changes will ensure your center remains compliant and financially sustainable.

6. **Embrace innovation and technology:** Adopt new technologies and innovative approaches to treatment that can enhance the client experience and improve outcomes. This may include incorporating telehealth services, using data analytics to inform decision-making, or implementing new therapeutic modalities.

7. **Foster a culture of compassion and inclusion:** Create a welcoming and inclusive environment that values diversity and respects the unique experiences of each client and staff member. This can contribute to a positive atmosphere and promote healing for clients from all backgrounds.

Another key factor in the long-term success of your intensive outpatient treatment center is the ability to adapt to the evolving needs of clients and the healthcare industry. As new research emerges and treatment approaches evolve, your center must be able to stay ahead of the curve and provide cutting-edge care that meets the highest standards of quality.

To achieve this level of excellence, consider implementing the following practices:

1. **Encourage ongoing education and professional development:** Foster a culture of learning among staff members by providing regular training opportunities, continuing education courses, and access to research and industry publications. This can help keep staff members up to date on the latest advances in treatment and equip them with the skills and knowledge necessary to provide the highest quality care.

2. **Stay engaged with the community:** Regularly participate in community events and forums to stay abreast of local trends and needs. Building relationships with community leaders and stakeholders can also help raise awareness of your center's services and attract new clients.

3. **Leverage data to improve outcomes:** Use data analytics and other metrics to monitor client outcomes, track staff performance, and identify opportunities for improvement. This can help inform quality improvement initiatives and ensure that your center is delivering the most effective and efficient care possible.

4. **Foster a culture of innovation:** Encourage staff members to think creatively and embrace new ideas and technologies.

Regularly assess your center's operations and explore opportunities to improve efficiency and enhance the client experience through innovative approaches.

5. **Emphasize collaboration and communication:** Create a culture of collaboration and open communication among staff members, clients, and stakeholders. This can help build trust and promote a shared sense of purpose and responsibility for the well-being of clients.

By implementing these practices, your intensive outpatient treatment center can stay ahead of the curve and deliver the highest quality care possible. By prioritizing ongoing education and professional development, engaging with the community, leveraging data, fostering innovation, and emphasizing collaboration and communication, you can build a culture of excellence that makes a lasting impact on the lives of those you serve.

In addition to the practices outlined above, it is also essential to regularly assess and evaluate your center's operations to identify opportunities for improvement and ensure that your services are meeting the needs of your clients.

Consider implementing the following strategies to regularly assess and evaluate your center's operations:

1. **Conduct regular client satisfaction surveys:** Ask clients to provide feedback on their experience with your center, including

the effectiveness of treatment, the quality of care, and the overall client experience.

2. **Monitor client outcomes:** Use data analytics to track client outcomes, including rates of relapse, completion of treatment, and improvement in symptoms. Use this information to make data-driven decisions about how to improve your services and deliver the best possible outcomes for your clients.

3. **Assess staff performance:** Regularly evaluate staff members' performance through performance evaluations, peer reviews, and other methods. Use this information to identify areas where staff members may need additional training or support and to ensure that all staff members are providing high-quality care.

4. **Conduct regular audits:** Regularly audit your center's financial and operational processes to ensure that they are efficient, effective, and compliant with all applicable regulations and standards.

Another important aspect of running a successful intensive outpatient treatment center is fostering a culture of compassion, empathy, and support. Clients who come to your center may be struggling with serious mental health or substance use disorders and may feel vulnerable and in need of a supportive environment where they can feel safe and valued.

To create a culture of compassion and support, consider implementing the following strategies:

1. **Create a welcoming environment:** Design your center's physical space to be warm, inviting, and comfortable. Use calming colors, natural light, and comfortable furnishings to create a space that feels safe and welcoming to clients.

2. **Hire staff who embody your values:** When hiring staff members, look for individuals who share your center's values of compassion, empathy, and support. Consider behavioral-based interviewing techniques to identify candidates who have a demonstrated commitment to these values.

3. **Provide ongoing training in empathy and communication skills:** Ensure that all staff members receive training in empathy and effective communication skills. This can help them build strong relationships with clients, understand their needs, and respond appropriately to their concerns.

4. **Foster a sense of community:** Create opportunities for clients to connect with one another and form a sense of community within your center. This can help clients feel less isolated and more supported during the recovery process.

5. **Encourage client participation in their own care:** Empower clients to take an active role in their own care by providing them with information, resources, and opportunities to make decisions about their treatment. This can help clients feel more invested in their recovery and more confident in their ability to achieve their goals.

Another important aspect of operating a successful intensive outpatient treatment center is staying up to date with the latest research, treatment approaches, and best practices in the field. The field of mental health and substance use treatment is constantly evolving, and staying informed about new developments and trends can help you deliver the best possible care to your clients.

Consider implementing the following strategies to stay informed about the latest research and best practices:

1. **Attend professional development opportunities:** Attend conferences, workshops, and other professional development opportunities to stay up to date with the latest research and trends in the field. This can help you gain new insights, expand your knowledge base, and connect with other professionals in the industry.

2. **Read professional journals and publications:** Subscribe to professional journals and publications related to mental health and substance use treatment. This can help you stay informed about the latest research, best practices, and emerging trends in the field.

3. **Participate in peer review and supervision:** Participate in peer review and supervision sessions with other mental health and substance use treatment professionals. This can help you gain feedback on your own work, share knowledge with others in the field, and stay informed about new developments and best practices.

4. **Collaborate with other healthcare providers:** Build relationships with other healthcare providers in your community, including primary care physicians, psychiatrists,

and other specialists. This can help you stay informed about the latest research and trends in the field, and provide your clients with a comprehensive network of support.

Another important aspect of running a successful intensive outpatient treatment center is maintaining a commitment to ethical and professional conduct. As a provider of mental health and substance use treatment, your center has a responsibility to operate in a manner that upholds the highest standards of ethical and professional behavior.

Consider implementing the following strategies to ensure that your center maintains a commitment to ethical and professional conduct:

1. Develop and enforce a code of ethics: Develop a code of ethics that outlines the ethical principles and values that guide your center's operations. Ensure that all staff members are aware of the code of ethics, and enforce it consistently and fairly.

2. Maintain confidentiality and privacy: Ensure that all client information is kept confidential and secure, in compliance with relevant laws and regulations. Establish clear policies and procedures for maintaining confidentiality, and ensure that all staff members are trained in these policies and procedures.

3. Avoid conflicts of interest: Ensure that your center avoids conflicts of interest that could compromise the quality or integrity of care provided to clients. Develop policies and

procedures to address potential conflicts of interest, and ensure that all staff members are trained in these policies and procedures.

4. Provide informed consent: Ensure that all clients provide informed consent before beginning treatment. This includes providing clients with information about their treatment options, the risks and benefits of treatment, and their rights and responsibilities as clients.

5. Implement regular quality assurance and improvement measures: Implement regular quality assurance and improvement measures to ensure that your center is delivering the highest quality care to clients. This can include monitoring client outcomes, conducting regular client satisfaction surveys, and reviewing policies and procedures to identify areas for improvement.

By maintaining a commitment to ethical and professional conduct, your center can build a reputation as a trusted and effective provider of mental health and substance use treatment. This can help attract new clients through positive word-of-mouth and ensure that your center delivers the highest quality care to clients.

Another important aspect of running a successful intensive outpatient treatment center is creating a positive and supportive organizational culture. The culture of your center can have a significant impact on the quality of care provided to clients, as well as the job satisfaction and retention of staff members.

Consider implementing the following strategies to create a positive and supportive organizational culture:

1. **Foster a culture of collaboration and teamwork:** Encourage collaboration and teamwork among staff members and create opportunities for staff members to work together on shared goals and projects. This can help build a sense of community and shared purpose among staff members.

2. **Provide ongoing training and professional development:** Provide ongoing training and professional development opportunities to staff members, and support their growth and development as professionals. This can help staff members feel valued and invested in the success of the center.

3. **Promote work-life balance:** Promote work-life balance among staff members, and provide opportunities for staff members to take breaks and recharge throughout the day. This can help prevent burnout and promote overall well-being.

4. **Recognize and reward staff members for their contributions:** Recognize and reward staff members for their contributions to the center, and create a culture of appreciation and gratitude. This can help build a positive and supportive work environment and promote job satisfaction and retention among staff members.

Finally, just have fun. Having fun in your business is an often overlooked but important aspect of running a successful intensive outpatient treatment center. While the focus of your center is on providing high-quality mental health and substance use treatment, it is also important to create a positive and enjoyable work environment for staff members and clients.

Consider implementing the following strategies to create an enjoyable environment at your center:

1. **Plan regular team building activities:** Plan regular team building activities that allow staff members to connect and have fun together outside of work. This can include activities such as group outings, team-building exercises, and social events.

2. **Incorporate fun into daily operations:** Find ways to incorporate fun and humor into daily operations at your center. This can include decorating the center with colorful and engaging artwork, playing upbeat music in common areas, or incorporating games and activities into therapy sessions.

3. **Celebrate successes and milestones:** Celebrate successes and milestones at your center, and create opportunities for staff members and clients to recognize and celebrate each other's achievements. This can help build a positive and supportive community at your center.

4. **Create a welcoming and inviting environment:** Create a welcoming and inviting environment at your center that feels warm and inviting. This can include providing comfortable seating and amenities such as coffee and snacks for clients and

creating a visually appealing and calming space for therapy sessions.

By incorporating fun and enjoyment into your daily operations and creating a welcoming and inviting environment, your center can build a positive and supportive community that promotes healing and recovery.

I sincerely hope that this guidebook has provided you with valuable insights and practical strategies for opening and operating a successful intensive outpatient treatment center. If you found it helpful, please consider leaving a positive review on Amazon. Positive reviews not only help us but also make it easier for other potential readers to find the book and benefit from its contents.

Our team has invested a great deal of effort and expertise in creating a guidebook that is up-to-date, practical, and informative. We understand the challenges involved in running a successful treatment program, and we are committed to helping you overcome them.

In closing, I wish you the best of luck in your journey to provide compassionate care to those struggling with addiction and mental illness. By using the insights and strategies provided in this guidebook, you can make a positive difference in the lives of your patients and their families.

Thank you for considering this guidebook, and I hope that you have found it informative, insightful, and practical.

-R. Cord Beatty

www.ingramcontent.com/pod-product-compliance
Lightning Source LLC
Chambersburg PA
CBHW051205220625
28556CB00009B/321